- Tantric Sex -

The Ultimate Step by Step Guide to Tantric Sex
for Couples with Tantric Sex Positions,
Tantric Massage, Yoga & Meditation

By

Madison Streep

2020 © Copyright

Introduction

The originally stormy sex life of couples begins to settle down after being together for a while. All the interesting poses from the Kama Sutra have been tried, sex games have been played. You got stuck in a routine and want new sensations? Maybe it's time to try something fundamentally new? Then go ahead! Read this book and you will find out how to practice Tantric sex and what Tantra is. Tantric sex is a special kind of love that allows you and your partner to get to know each other even better and get an unearthly pleasure. Believe me, the game is worth the candle, you just need to do everything right!

Generally, tantric sex is part of the unique philosophical system that came to us from India. This type of intimacy implies not that much physical, but rather the obligatory spiritual union of the partners. During such sex, the kundalini energy (sexual energy), sleeping in the lowest chakras, awakens and rises up to the head, through the energy channel in the spine. We offer you in this book a detailed, clearly defined program for understanding and practicing Tantric Sex at best.

This book will help you to reveal the intricacies, secrets of Tantra and learn specific exercises to transform your sexuality into the spiritual fire of love and bliss of true unity with your partner. By reading this book you will discover Tantric meditation methods and how to transform the loving act from animal instinct into a spiritual and evolutionary practice. You will go through the exciting adventure exploring Mantras, Yantras and Mandalas. This book will open to you a wide variety of Tantric Sex positions, which will bring novelty to your sex life, expanding the range of available sensations previously unthinkable. You will learn how to heat up your bedroom with Tantric massage and explore Tantric Yoga, which will help you to unleash your sexual energy. In this book you will discover this and much more. So what are you waiting for, start reading and enjoying!

Table of Contents

Copyright, Legal Notice And Disclaimer

Disclaimer Notice

Please note that the information contained within this document is for educational and entertainment purpose only. Every attempt has been made to provide accurate, up to date and reliable complete information. No warranties of any kind are expressed or implied. Readers acknowledge that the author is not engaging in the rendering of legal, financial, medical or professional advice.

Please consider consulting a licensed professional before attempting any techniques outlined in this book. By reading this document, the readers agree that under no circumstances are we responsible for any losses, direct or indirect, which are incurred as results of the use of information contained within this document, including, but not limited to, errors, omission, or inaccuracies.

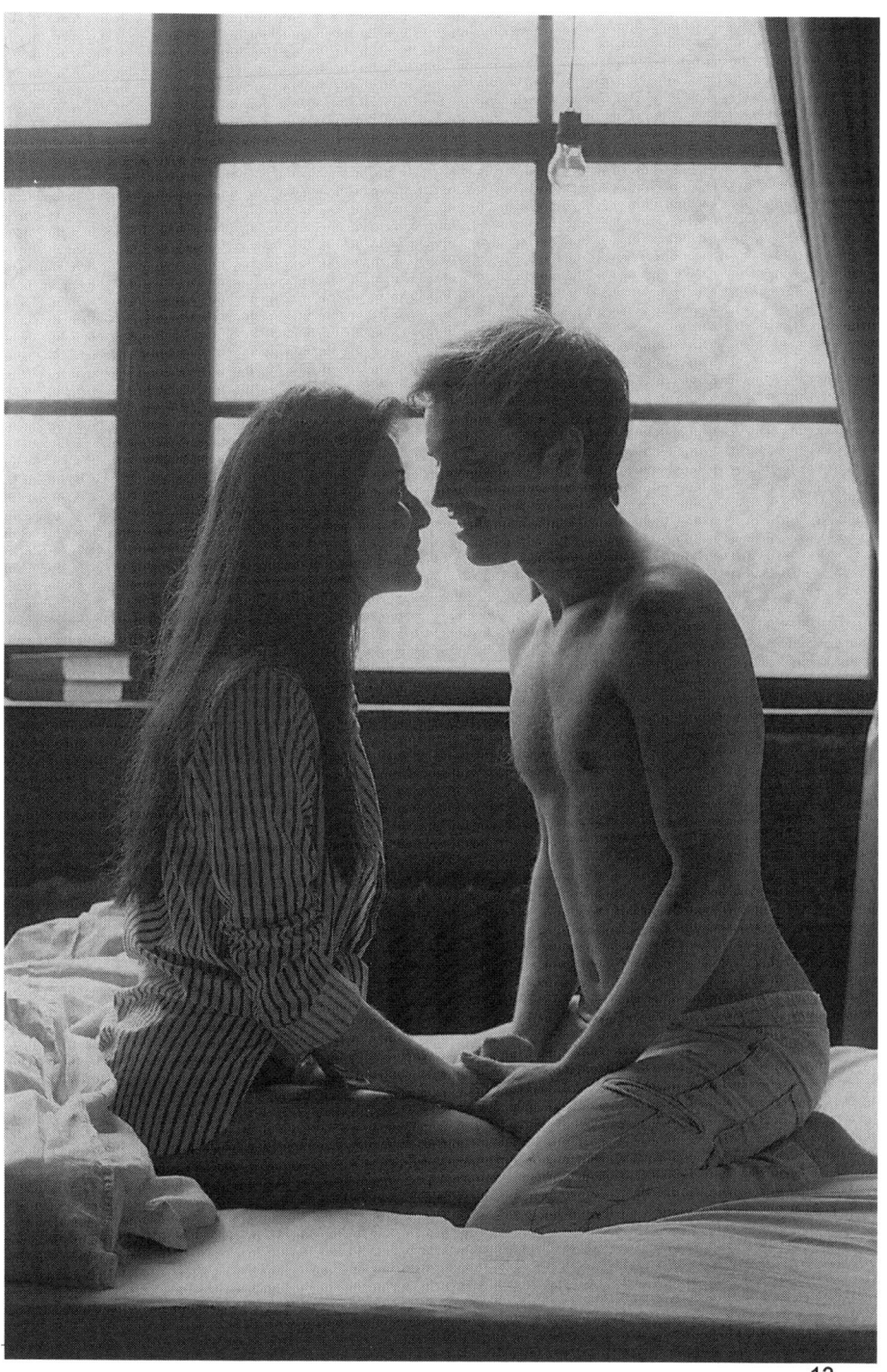

Chapter 1: Tantra, Getting Started

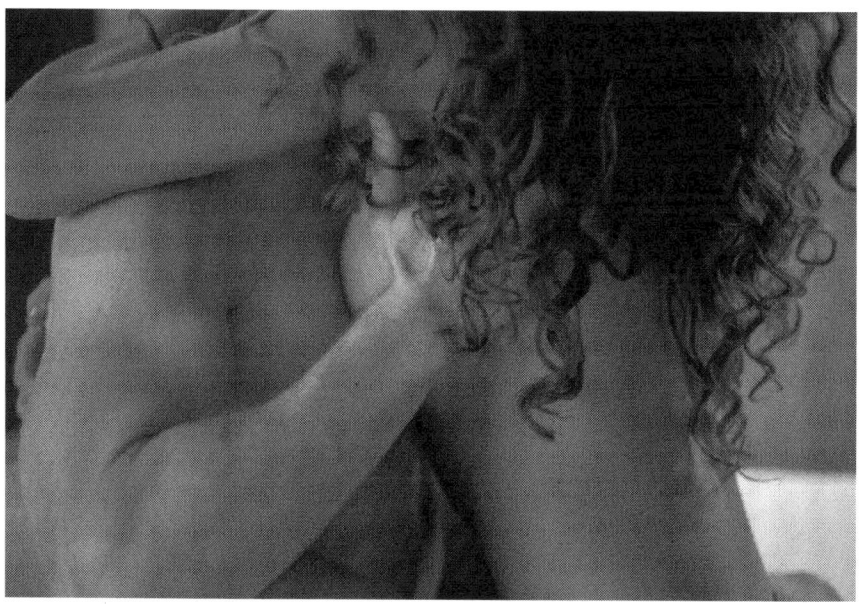

Tantra is a philosophy of life and self-care that involves yoga, meditation, sex, diet and massage.

What is Tantra

The word Tantra originates from Sanskrit, and is composed of the root Tan = "extend, multiply", and the suffix Tra = "tool and liberation". It is a set of millenary doctrines and practices aimed at expanding the ordinary state of consciousness. Tantric yoga, tantric massage, tantric meditation: these are closely related practices. They refer to all those tools that are developed to extend human consciousness. The evocative image of the fabric, produced with the loom through the weaving of warp and weft, represents the metaphor of the union of individual and universal consciousness, and of the male with the female.

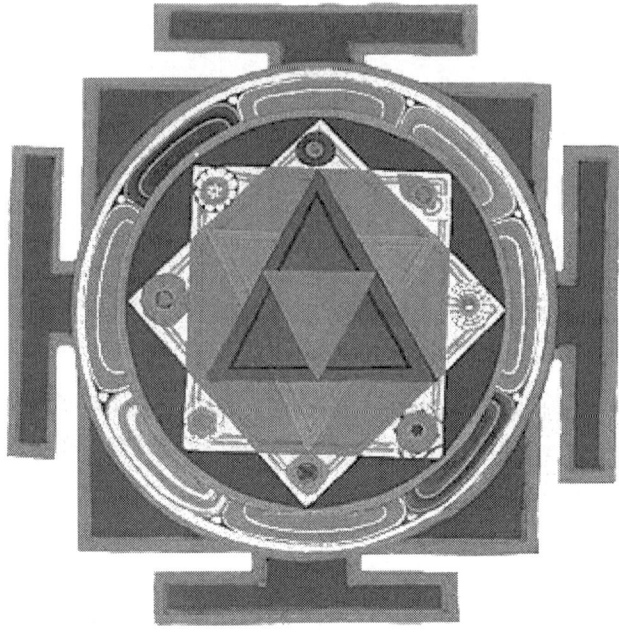

Tantra is therefore a process to make us more conscious. It pushes us to awaken us, to be more attentive to the restrictions and identifications of our false ego and to transform the masks with which we also use our sexual energy and become more vital through the transmission and crossing of all our energies that make us up: transcendent energy, mental energy, expressive energy, affective energy, radiant energy, emotional energy and sexual energy.

Tantric philosophy has roots both in archaic Buddhism and Hinduism, the oldest Tantra (philosophical reference texts) are of Buddhist compilation and date back to 350 AD. At the center of Tantric thought there is the "manifest" universe, considered as physical expression and sensorial of the "unmanifest": hence the idea that, through immersion in the former, one can achieve full unity with the latter. To achieve this it is necessary to follow a very rigid discipline which, however, varies depending on the practitioner's level of consciousness. All levels have in common the work on the harmonization of male and female energy, Shiva and Shakty, which are reminiscent of the Taoist Ying and Yang, and the aim is to appropriately awaken and channel the Kundalini energy, the custodian of the secret of 'lighting".

How does it work

Asana, mantra, pranayama, meditation and right actions, are the truly fundamental components of Tantra, and these are the elements that are mixed in the different schools. Each school differs from the others because it shifts the emphasis on one or the other.

In the tantric path, the so-called "right hand" and "left hand" ways are clearly distinguished. In the schools of the right hand the precepts that drive the union of the male and female principle are interpreted as a metaphor for the union at an energy level, while in the ways of the left hand they are literally interpreted. Hence originates maithuna - the secret ritual of love - which is not however a central practice, although Tantra is today commonly associated with this. On the contrary maithuna is considered one of the highest and last stages that the yogi must face because only true yogis can afford to practice it as a meditation technique.

In the physical field, the benefits of tantra yoga are those specific to any other form of yoga, and vary according to which elements the school prefers. In the case of schools that favor the physical aspect (Hatha, Iyengar, Power etc.), the greatest benefits will come from the spine, the musculoskeletal system, the lengthening of the tendons and the looseness of the joints. Therefore they will dissolve and soothe contractures, tensions, joint and muscle pains. In the case of schools that favor the meditative-energetic aspect (Kundalini), the benefits will involve the psychological dimension with a marked improvement in mood, decrease in stress, containment of depressive states, an increase in the ability to concentrate.

Undoubtedly the tantric approach helps to alleviate the tensions of the couple, bringing benefits in case of problems in the intimate relationship and when eventual couples' issues have psychological roots. All thanks to the relaxed and non-competitive approach to the intimate relationship where all tension from "performance anxiety" decays.

Why is Tantra useful

In recent times Tantra has experienced great fame in the West, mainly due to the mistakenly emphasis placed on the use of certain sexual practices; these actually constitute only a part of the tantric doctrine; the tantric doctrine combines body and mind, joy and spirituality, the recognition of the sacredness of Life, a solid moral basis, the daily practice of Asanas for the purification of the body and energy channels, exercises of concentration and meditation. The Tantric dimension of yogic practice is therefore designed for all those who wish to deepen their physical-spirit-mind relationship thanks to yoga, meditation and specific exercises to make the energetic perception even more subtle.

The Tantra yoga is one of the most well-known forms of yoga, taught and practiced in the West: Kundalini yoga, Hatha yoga,

Raja yoga, Laya yoga and Mantra yoga. In all these tantric yoga schools, priority is given to practices and rituals of a mainly physical type. Tantra is practiced and considered more a philosophy of life than a type of proper cure in the West. We remember that the holistic operator is a professional capable of carrying out manuals treatments of energy aimed at rebalancing, restoration, maintaining and boosting vitality and psychophysical well-being, therefore improving the quality of life.

Tantric practice builds and demolishes reality, like a game, until it becomes the true nature of things, the essence, the pure potential that explodes in energy and matter at all times. The tantric practitioner shatters the ordinary appearance by creating new existential structures. It is not a question of creative visualizations in the generally used sense, but of deconstructing blocks of reality and reconstructing other alternatives. The goal is to recognize one's own intimate, intrinsic primordial nature in all appearances.

It is the way of ecstasy that through the use also of sexual energy, the most powerful force we have, allows us to experience the body as a sacred space in which ardor, the flame of sex is expressed.

When the true nature of everything is revealed, even the most insignificant moment acquires extreme beauty that shakes the mind. In this way, there is nothing more ordinary in life. Tantra encourages you to live life intensely, totally, freeing it from tensions, pre-established models, inhibitions. It is the path of the soul that also honors the body by celebrating the senses and life experiences. It is saying yes to vitality, to the sacredness of the body and to the joy of sexuality and love.

Tantra is the practice that uses sex only as a medium, in a healing context of love for oneself and others. In short, nothing to do with the intent to take control of one's sexual performance, even if this can happen very often as a secondary effect, due to a greater knowledge of ourselves and our reactions.

Our civilization has historically prohibited the expression of love by condemning sexuality, the contemporary world ignores love while exploiting sexuality, the tantric must break these stereotypes and challenge moral precepts because sex represents the mean through which we can reach to know love. Love is transformed sexual energy.

Emotions and passions in Tantra

In Tantra, desires, emotions and passions have a powerfully creative role and are considered the means that, through sensoriality, leads to the Self, the most authentic and free part of us: for this reason it is called "the way of pleasure". It is a way that opposes hedonistic research, generalized materialism, romantic supernaturalism and religious fundamentalisms, since it unifies sensoriality and awareness, sensuality and spirituality in a subtle and profound approach.

Tantra is also called Vama Marga or "the way of the left hand" because the woman, who represents the lunar influence, the negative or left polarity, plays an essential role in this way. However, the way recommended here is not made up of negativity and austerity as in most other spiritual systems, but is a way of acceptance, pleasure and bliss. Tantric tradition clearly shows that the state of harmonious integration and spiritual freedom can be obtained through direct experience and living everyday life. The lower levels of consciousness cannot be controlled without effort and overcome without being fully and frantically lived, intensely and totally, in the fullness of their powers.

The term Tantra summarizes the notions of Liberation and Expansion: it is, in practice, a sacred science that allows access to the Absolute (Brahma), through techniques of psychic and bodily expansion that also, but not exclusively, concern eros individual, couple or group. It is a metaphysics that allows, if followed with the help of the study of traditional texts and a qualified teaching, to get out of the individual sphere, from the world as we normally understand it, and to follow itineraries that free from conditioning and limitations, first the psyche, then the spiritual mind, finally the entire cosmos, when you are able to identify yourself and everything around you.

The goal of Tantra is to make each of us discover out our true and intrinsic nature, getting rid of all the limits and the masks we have. Mind and body come together as in a dance and from this derives a great sense of well-being and awareness.

Merging sensory, emotional and cognitive levels with spiritual

Tantra has the characteristic of merging the sensory, emotional and cognitive levels with the spiritual one and of relying on the recognition and integration of polarities (male / female, active / passive, eroticism / meditation, control / ecstasy). In addition to creating a bridge between sexuality and spirit, Tantra connects two directions of spiritual research which are kept separate in other schools: Control and Ecstasy. In Tantra the object of research is mainly that vibration of consciousness that brings together these opposite poles of subjective experience, along two paths, the active and the passive one, which are both practiced by the "Tantrists".

When a participant reaches a higher stage of awareness, through the control of the vital energy it also becomes possible to use sex to promote spiritual growth.

Tantra love

Tantra offers a series of gradual psycho-spiritual techniques for the development and experience of genuine love. Love that does not invite the renunciation of desire, but rather seeks its refinement and transcendence, and in the trance of the mystical union invites to travel towards beauty and pleasure, knowing that only a satisfied body can open itself to higher experiences. The body is in fact an essential tool, without which evolution itself would be practically impossible. If the problems of survival, mental and physical well-being have not been solved, inner peace is not achieved. We must therefore not forget that the two aspects, material and spiritual, are not mutually exclusive, but on the contrary they are never clearly separable from each other.

It is the exact opposite of asceticism. According to tantric doctrines, the body is the mean by which the spirit can rise. The opposite of abstinence practices, that conceive the body as the first enemy of the spirit.

Tantrism is the way that best suits the man who lives in this age which is not that of pure detachment, but that of knowledge, of awakening, of the domain of secret energies contained in the body. Tantra, in fact, does not aim to give up the world, but to feel it with fullness and integrity. For too many centuries the life of the spirit and the ordinary and of the body have been unjustly kept apart. Tantra ends this dichotomy.

Tantra is not coercive and no text tries to proselytize. Free membership is considered a fundamental request and spontaneous consent is the only way through which the tantric mystery can be accessed. For this reason, the consent of the person with whom to complete the incredible path of the tantric path is essential.

It is possible to really meet, in a space of reconciliation where women and men can learn about their diversity and find within them those tools that help to discover meeting points.

It starts from accepting yourself, from loving yourself and from allowing yourself to meet others in pleasure. Tantra integrates your sexuality, your emotions, senses and awareness, bringing you into a state of meditation, of abandonment.

The Tantra path

Tantra is a path of self-discovery, a path of joy. You need to be extremely honest with your inner dynamics, and not everyone is willing to strip naked in such a way.

The body in Tantra is in fact considered the temple of the divine (sacred reality) and is seen as the microcosm where the individual soul resides in order to understand the macrocosm of the Universe. The body is a mystical symbol for tantrics, only a vehicle with which to experience in this life and which assists us in the process of spiritual growth and in the process of acquiring the experience itself. Without energy and sensitivity in the body and without proper use we cannot go far towards enlightenment. In the body there is a cosmic intelligence that guides us and manifests itself when we no longer use the body following our personal desires but using it as a tool for developing higher awareness.

In Tantra, the meeting with the partner stimulates sexual energy, called kundalini, to expand and rise along the chakras, "energy centers" of the body. At the same time, the meditative attitude - that is, of observation, presence and understanding - allows the energy of the spiritual planes to descend into the body itself. Therefore, the two energies, linked respectively to earth and sky, meet within the human being (at the height of the vital center corresponding to the heart) and it is said that man experiences within himself his own "woman inner ", and the woman of her" inner man ". This is a fusion experience that transcends the ordinary state of separation in which the human being lives.

Love, passion and desire are born "magically" in the encounter between man and woman. However, as daily experience shows, these fundamental ingredients of the couple often end up fading, leading to boredom and disenchantment. Tantra sheds light on the emotional dynamics of life for two and also proposes solutions to get out of the routine and actively culti-vate, over the years, love and passion.

A sexual relationship can elevate or "empty" us, make us feel dirty or give us profound joy, it depends on the type of energy that we put into it.

Man's ability to go beyond the vision of a mental world domi-nated by opposites and conflicts, to understand that he himself is the producer of this world, but also to have the ability to change it, to unite the opposites, to finally live in the joy and in perfect harmony with the true rhythms of nature. The race for success, for money, for power, for prevarication over one another, for the triumph of the ego are the real causes of frustrations, personality disorders, sexuality issues and depressions.

Tantra and sex

Thanks to Tantra it is possible to expand the perception of sexuality, transforming it into a divergent experience in which every cell of the body participates, and in which time in its common sense ceases to exist.

The tantric achieves this result by channeling the energy awakened by the practices by touching all the main energy centers (chackra) of the body during the ascent.

Tantra is therefore neither a philosophy, nor a religion, nor a discipline or a technique: it is a "way". This concept, unusual for the western mentality, indicates an experiential path, structured and conceived to lead the soul - the spiritual part of the human being - to reunite with the divine principle of the universe that the soul already contains within self and re-balance the forces of women and men through the use of the body, the vehicle that accompanies us throughout life. Sexuality, being however one of the most important and decisive experiences for a human being, is considered in Tantra an integral part in the personal and spiritual growth of an individual.

All sensations, all pleasures are therefore, after all, emanations of the Divine. The senses have the ability to experience delight and amazement and, therefore, the practitioner will use them to increase his awareness. If we raise the level of sensitivity towards the beauty of everything around us, we can get closer and closer to the sense of wonder and amazement emanating from creation, which is the uninterrupted pulsation of consciousness that pervades any experience.

Tantra trains to listening intimately and consciously of oneself and the other, also using sexuality as a vehicle to dissolve the resistances and conditioning of the Ego in ardor, and bring us to the deep and pure encounter of hearts, to meeting with the Primordial Energy that is within us.

Making sex a playful and sincere moment, a space to explore, enrich ourselves and the love act. When sex becomes a habitual performance generating anxiety and not relaxation, the natural pleasure it generates is blocked in both men and women.

The sex seen by us Westerners often resembles a test, a performance which, as such, requires competitiveness with oneself and with the partner. The transfer of competitiveness from life and work to the sexual sphere can be said to occur. The condemnation and repression that sex and the body have suffered over the centuries, especially in the West, have distorted their essence by depriving us of the joy that comes from the natural contact with ourselves.

We often forget that we were born from an orgasm and a healthy "eros" is a source of deep nourishment. Unfortunately, this nourishment is hindered by the many conditionings and fears that are poured out on ourselves by the family, society, religion, morals. This leads us to experience profound contradictions between the natural drive to pleasure, which is the birthright of the human race, and the conditions that create the ideal psychological places for the sense of guilt and shame. All this affects our life at the roots leading to a progressive loss of trust and self-esteem and limiting our ability to love.

The invitation of Tantra is simple: live sexuality with the fullness of the subtle senses that you have developed, rejoice in it in the fullness of perfumes, taste, vision and touch, drowned in the "here and now" of the intense pleasure that it causes you, and at the same time reminds you that the "samadhi" you feel (that is, the sense of fulfillment given by the fusion) is only the pale anticipation of a much higher samadhi that awaits you: the fusion with the whole.

According to Tantra, the sensation that can be experienced can be described as an experience in which the orgasm is of the whole body and runs through it completely, ending very gradually in a great ecstasy.

Sexuality experienced tantrically, therefore, is nothing but the finger that points to the moon. Only the fool gets lost looking at the finger: the target is the moon.

Once understood the meaning of sex as a symbol, the latter can also be abandoned, although tantra does not address any invitation to do so. Basically, as the great masters have well understood, once the conscience is freed from emotional dependence on sexuality, the latter can still be lived or not, with the freedom of those who have risen to a higher level and no longer come conditioned by the lower ones.

Through this way we will discover that Tantra is the map to awaken yourself, together with the other. How can this happen? The first step is contact with your body and that of your loved one. Our bodies are the temple. Tantra teaches you to have deep respect, gratitude, love. If contact with the body is lost contact with reality is lost.

But when you allow the body's energy to flow giving it total freedom, you are able to be totally in the other, to totally flow in the other. Thus the couple's relationship will be vital, the source of new creative processes and spiritual growth

Even today, Tantra appears profoundly revolutionary. Perhaps, precisely because it is so ancient that it cannot grow old. It is not a philosophy to be discussed, it is not a problem to be solved but a "mystery to bc lived" and a "space in which to exist", as indicated by the Indian philosopher and teacher Osho. Tantra urges to experience the flow of life totally and in first person, and in this it leaves no room for intermediaries.

Chapter 2: History Of Tantra

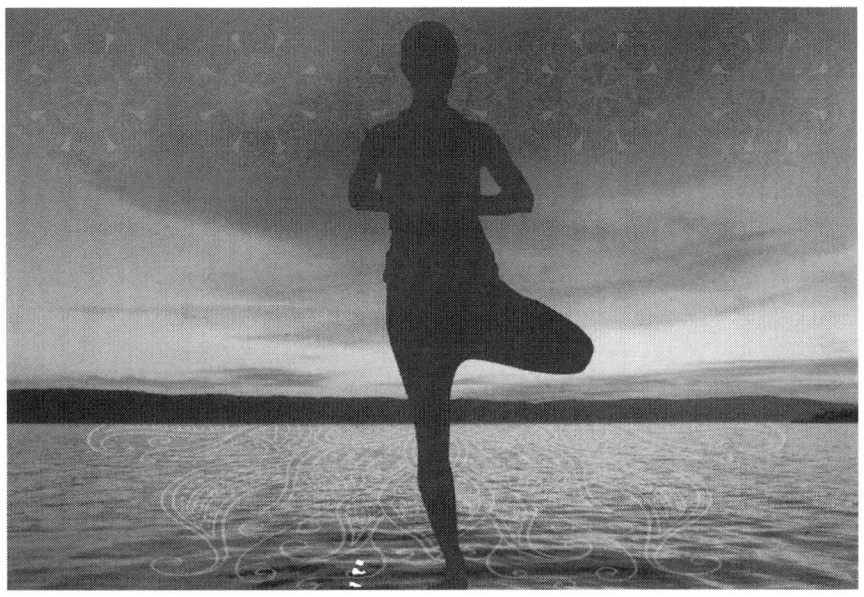

The original tantra, also called "red" or "left hand" is linked to ancient matriarchal societies and has female energy as its center. While the Tantra called "White" or "right-handed", created later due to Muslim infiltrations, derives from Indian patriarchal societies.

The difference between Red Tantra and White Tantra is radical. The second, White Tantra, is based on static and solitary meditations, while Red Tantra is a practice in which meditation is not just immobility and seriousness. In Red Tantra meditation and sacredness are experienced in every moment of existence, through deep listening and attention to what is happening in us and outside of us. Meditation occurs while dancing, working, embracing, eating, drinking, playing and talking.

There is a lot of confusion about what Tantra really is and above all a lot of targeted misinformation, due to the persecutions to which the Original Tantra was subjected. Tantra carries with it the burden of false commonplaces, such as that of free sex. Unlike other disciplines that have been less polluted, Tantra is for many a kind of Yoga practice; for others an orgiastic practice and for still others a religion.

The origin of Tantra

According to the almost unanimous opinion of scholars, the archaic nature of Red Tantra dates back to pre-Vedic cultures, to the very beginnings of Indian history, identifiable with the Harappei, Sindhu and other Dravidian populations who developed their civilization in the Indus valley. According to some in the third millennium BC these populations were widespread in a huge territory that went from Spain to the Ganges valley. Their precursors had settled in the Indus valley in Mehrgar starting from 7000 BC. and their traces can be found up to 5500 BC.

Dravidian populations, therefore, appeared there around 6000-5000 BC, had their apogee between 2300 and 1300 BC. and disappeared, rather quickly, in a 100-year period between 1900 and 1800 B.C. The reasons for the disappearance were attributed in the past to invasions of the Arii population from the north. Today there is a tendency to attribute it rather to a tectonic movement that caused the Aravali hills in northern Rajastan to rise, depriving the river that supported the Dravida civilization (the Ghaggar-Hakra) of most of its tributaries.

The Harappei population showed a marked interest in the arts and well-being. Theirs was a matriarchal society, the most important central monument of their city, it was a large swimming pool; the element of water was fundamental in their society and there has already been a bathroom in every home. The woman was at the center of culture, focused on the mother goddess. The female figure dominated the sanctuaries and with open arms and legs, offered herself to adoration. The Harappei used to keep a large bed in the center of the most important room in the house and practiced Tantra. Their religion was closely connected with the body, well-being and sexuality.

It can be said that Red Tantra is the expression of all those practices which also include sexuality. Red Tantra includes practices that are also carried out in groups, including contact and "vehiculation" through the senses.

In the centuries following the birth of Tantra, in India, due to the Islamic invasions, the original Red Tantra was officially suppressed and forced to transform itself into an occult school. Thus was born the White Tantra, which had monastic aspects and was without sexual intercourse; it was generally more tolerated but gradually lost its identity eventually merging with Yoga. Today we know it as Tantra Yoga, and it has completely lost its peculiarity of concrete approach to sexuality, typical of the original Tantra.

In practice the White Tantra is a Red Tantra but censored by all those practices that moralists could understand as unbecoming. Today the White Tantra, which is therefore a mystification of the original Tantra, is used in the West for commercial purposes. Almost all Tantra schools practice White Tantra and therefore do not actually teach Tantra.

True Tantra is the Way of reconnection with one's Self. It is the Way; that of the discovery of our genotypic sexual energies that are manifested through the knowledge and practice of the Original Tantra.

The Tantra texts

The Tantras are a series of texts of Central Asian origin (India, Kashmir, Bengal, Orissa, Assam, Kerala, Indus Valley etc.) like the collections of the Puranas or the Vedas, but which manifest themselves in the manner of esoteric texts divine revealed and are often written as if they were the gods Shiva and Shakty (and their emanations) in person speaking and are part of the Hindu texts Agama.

The origin of the Tantras is pre-Vedic, that is much older than the texts on which Hinduism and the Vedas are based, and originates from the ancient matriarchal peoples and in general all the collections of Hindu texts are deeply influenced by the Tantra. There is no Hindu and Brahmin ritual that does not have its roots in Tantra.

The Tantras were transcribed long after their birth, as previously the tradition was handed down only orally from master to teacher, from teacher to teacher. In fact, in Tantra, unlike Hinduism, the teachers could be men or women. Starting from about the VI AD instead the written transcriptions of many Tantras begin to appear.

Tantric texts have more than one reading and can be experienced at different levels of intuition. According to the Tantric tradition, a text can confuse or illuminate. Tantric texts often speak by aphorisms (sutra and karika) and often then generate immense commentaries that explain aphorisms that can sometimes be difficult to understand.

The term Tantra, linked to the ancient texts, was then translated also to indicate the Spiritual Experiential Way that follows these ancient teachings.

More than 500 existing Tantras are known which belong to different initiatory ways or lineages, (Aghora, Āḷvār, Bāul, Gauḍīya, Kālāmukha, Pāśupata, Sahajiyā, Śaivasiddhānta, Saura, Shakta, Spanda, Surya, Śrīvidyā, Trika, Kālīkula, Kānpaṭha, Kāpālika, Krama, Kaula, Lākula, Liṅgāyat, Nātha, Nāyaṇar, Pāñcarātra, etc.) and many of them have never even been translated from Sanskrit. Other tantric texts have been lost and it is not known what they handed down. It is said that the texts reached the considerable number of 14000 volumes. So the panorama of tantric initiatory texts is very vast and not all Tantras treat themes equally according to the lineage to which they belong. So this also generates some confusion regarding the teachings. Some Tantric Texts can be of few pages, others of thousands of pages.

It should therefore be understood that different teachings are grouped under the word Tantra, although on many points, many Tantra essentially agree. It cannot be said that the various tantric texts contradict each other, but that they simply give a certain importance more to one aspect than to another. Some Tantras favor the transmission of the concept of Presence, others of the concept of the Body, others with respect to Sexuality. A generally shared aspect is the "freed in life", that is, the unnecessary need for countless reincarnations to dissolve Karma. In fact, in tantra it is indicated that by following certain rituals or teachings it is possible to dissolve the karmic knots quickly, soon arriving at a knowledge of oneself also through the experimentation of eros and sexuality in the encounter between Shiva and Shakti and in any case following a way away from the renunciation of the body.

The revelations of the Tantras are considered superior to the Vedas because they are much more effective in the liberation of men and lead them faster to a higher stage and are more suitable for the current cosmic era, the Kaliyuga. Tantra considers the Vedic texts to be valid, but on a lower level as basic general rules, but which are then integrated by higher and esoteric specific tantric teachings.

Tantric texts do not address the renunciating ascetic of the world, but on the contrary they address those who live in the world, together with others, without going away or dedicating themselves to asceticism.

How did Tantra arrive in the west

In conjunction with the sexual liberation of the 60s and 70s and the emancipation of women, some scholars and philosophers began to talk about Tantra and trying to make it a practicable approach even in the West, made the rituals more agile and less blocking in the calculation of breathe and holding of positions. Currently emancipation allows women to get closer to the sexual world, although in western society it is still believed that sex is more masculine than feminine and cultural heritage does not allow women to focus on that.

In the West today Tantra aims to draw two maps, one that indicates how to make the sexual experience spiritual and how to unite the earth with the sky, in a terrain where separation and judgment vanish. A world, the western one, where there are no schools and traditions and everything is to be invented and experimented. In the West, the sexual sphere has been a world crushed for two millennia, by taboos and religions, which often finds its only expression in private clubs or porn sites.

Tantra and the way of liberation

Tantra with all its erotic experiences is nothing more than a tool that opens up internal physical, emotional and energetic spaces and opens up to awareness. Tantra is therefore only Red Tantra. It is the way of liberation that opens up to the true expression of one's self and that allows one to exit, both in the imaginary and in the real, from the dimension of the matrix in which sexual energy is mechanically channeled for improper purposes.

Sex and sexual energy are very different things. The idea of sex is what in the imagination has settled during education, stories and commercial pornography; a program therefore, but so rooted that individuals believe that it is precisely that pre-programmed way that sexual energy must be expressed. A program that is then gradually enhanced with the repetitive experiences that add up as memories.

The vital energy or commonly known as sexual energy (Kundalini), is instead what is really the essence of man at its origin; it is what we carry in our genes, but which due to the education received in the matrix, is then expressed in the facts in an unnatural way.

Over time, with the help of religious morality, the matrix selected a sexual modality aimed entirely at procreation, therefore mechanical and centered on penetration and orgasm intended as a goal to be achieved; as if all the wonder of the contact between the bodies should be enclosed in an act of a few minutes, between the two genital organs. Many people believe they are sexually free because they do a lot of that mechanical sex, while in reality they are just more slaves; slaves to a trap where true sexual energy is humiliated and crushed.

The true expression of sexual energy is in every moment we love something, a flower, a sunset or a caress. And when that energy expresses itself released from the mechanisms inculcated in the mind, it becomes ritual, celebration, connection of bodies, transcendence, healing energy, non-verbal communication, openness to trust between souls, breaking of mechanical schemes, projection into reality and into imaginary of a world made of love. Because love cannot be sought, love is a fruit of the tree of freedom. It is therefore freedom to generate love and it is precisely by freeing oneself from the patterns that love is encountered.

Chapter 3: Mantra

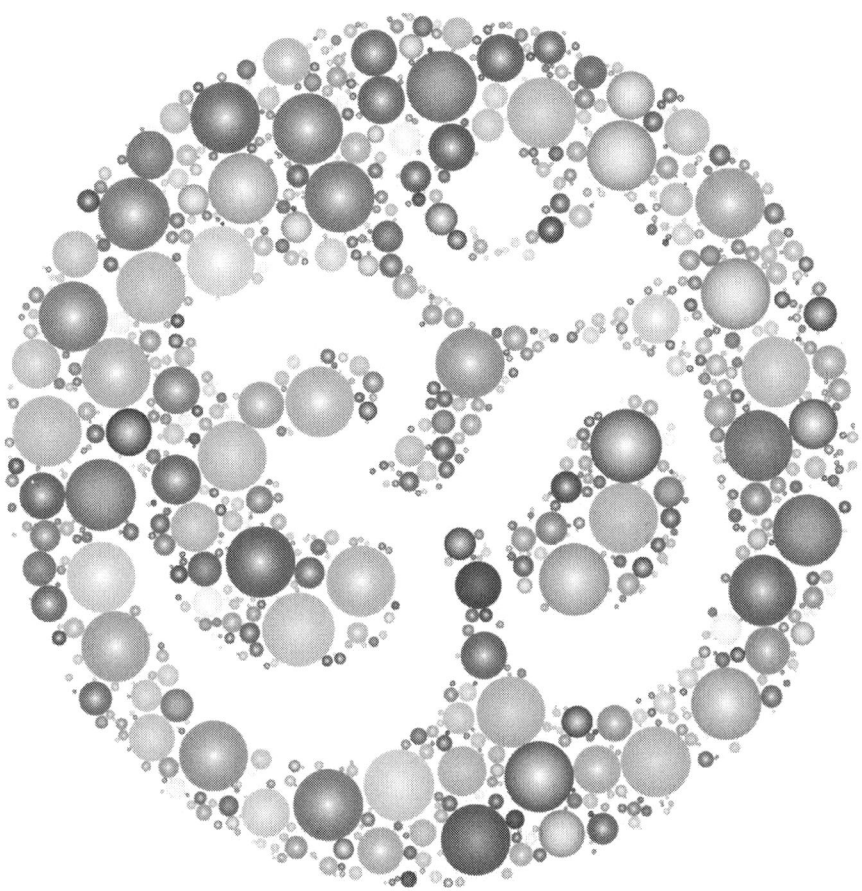

What is Mantra

Mantra is one of the most usually adopted tools in meditation, and also one of the most effective. The use of mantra meditation is established in many of the meditative traditions around the world and has a history old of many centuries.

Mantra is a Sanskrit word which comes from two source words: man, which means "mind" or "thinking", and trai, which means "protect", "free from" or "tool". Hence mantras are mind's tools, or better said tools for freeing the mind.

It is a word, or a sequence of words, designed to make our meditation more effective and bring numerous benefits on a spiritual level.

Some mantras incorporate a real meaning, but the majority according to belief, get their significance mainly from the type of sound. Some are small, 1-syllable mantras; others are longer and made of several words.

At times the mantra is recited, in other cases it is heard. Sometimes it must be repeated quickly, sometimes slowly. In certain situations it is simply recited alone, and at other times it is related to concentration, breath, chakras, visualization, or abstract thoughts. The mantras and the practices related to them are many and have their roots in Hinduism, yoga and Buddhism.

Why use a Mantra

The concept is actually very simple: sound is a pressure wave which is created by a vibrating object. The cells in the body vibrate. All in the universe is vibrant and all follows its own frequency. Thoughts and feelings are, in effect, the vibrations of your consciousness and your body. Sound waves also impact the water in the body, hormone production, thought, behavior and the wellbeing of the psyche.

Viewed from this point of view, your brain - your soul, mind, or spirit.- is a set of sounds, each pulsating at its own frequency, velocity and intensity. What the spiritualists and yogis have been able to discover is that by nourishing a particular sound for a prolonged time, the mind and body can be altered in some way, even temporarily.

Each musician or director is able to confirm the incredible power of sounds and their ability to influence moods, feelings and even what the person is thinking. If paying attention to a song can alter the way you feel and also aid to improve your body, try to think the impact of planning an ad-hoc sound in your mind, reiterating it several times with constancy and focus!

"Sound, rhythm and vocalizations have profound impact on the body, thoughts and feelings. Mantra meditation is the use of those components for the objective of cleaning, calming and altering your thoughts and soul."

Hence the Mantra, being a tool of the mind, can support in bringing deep changes in your body, soul, mind, or spirit and yield modified conditions of consciousness. Mantra meditation is a way of focusing your consciousness into a sound, intensifying it to get the best benefits. In the contemplative tradition, mantra meditation is considered the simplest and harmless method of obtaining deep benefits.

The Most known Mantra

The cosmic sound AUM (OM) is the origin of all the other sounds and is at the same time a Mantra. It is called Pranava, the sacred syllable, and symbolizes Brahman, the spiritual reality. It is the vibration emitted by Brahman that, by condensing the energy, created matter and the whole universe. The AUM Mantra leads to enlightenment. The chanting of the Om purifies the mind, destroys negativity and selfishness. AUM represents the trinity of body, mind and soul.

The flute of Lord Krishna also symbolizes Pranava. Through the sound of his flute, Krishna creates the world, and with his sound, he calls upon his devotees. Like the flute, the devotee must be empty, without selfishness and attachments. In this state of complete abandonment, the individual self merges with the universal Self and joy and harmony are experienced.

Mantra Yoga

Mantra Yoga is a part of Nada Yoga, the yoga of sound, and is only one of about 40 different approaches to Yoga. Nada Yoga consists of the theory and understanding of sound, vibration and music. Yogis have used the principles of Nada Yoga to align with the harmony of the universe. Mantra chanting is called Mantra Yoga.

Different forms of Mantra repetition are indicated with the term Japa Yoga, which can be:

- Vaikhari Japa if the Mantra is repeated aloud
- Upamsu Japa if the mantra is whispered
- Manasika Japa if repetition is mental
- Likhita Japa if the mantra is written.

The use of Mantra in any of these forms is effective in ensuring the concentration of the mind on a single point. Singing a Mantra with devotion and concentration has a harmonious influence on the whole body and mind. Concentration gives a sense of deep peace and joy, as can also happen with other forms of meditation. Through the constant repetition of the Mantra, its spiritual power is attracted, awareness is raised to the level of "mantric" resonance.

Mantra is a condensate of power that is activated by the intention of the one who practices it. When one begins the practice of a Mantra one must ask oneself what one wants to achieve, observe our mind during the practice (for this reason it is suggested to keep a spiritual diary).

The choice of Mantra is extremely important, because you get more results with a Mantra that you can completely abandon yourself to.

There are several ways in which you can choose a mantra (attraction, Guru, dream ...). After choosing or receiving a Mantra, one must persist in practice until one experiences its power. You have to resist the temptation to change it, thinking you have made the wrong choice, out of boredom or because the higher notes are difficult to reach.

They are the justifications of the mind that opposes to discipline and resists change. If you start with a Mantra, it is best to insist on the practice and build a good foundation.

In the practice of Japa, a mala is used to help count the repetitions. A mala is a necklace of 108 pearls, traditionally of sandalwood, tulsi (Indian basil) or rudraska seeds (they represent Shiva's tears of compassion for humans). 108 is a sacred number:

- The number 1, the line, symbolizes God, the energy, the power from which all other lines, circles or movements derive
- The 0 is a circle representing the creation of God as complete and perfect.
- The number 8 is the symbol of infinity.

At the point where the mala is tied, there is a special pearl, called Monte Meru. When you get to this pearl, you should turn the mala around and continue in the opposite direction. This pearl represents the divine realization and every time it is touched it should be remembered that it is no longer necessary for us to continue the chain of cause / effect that still holds us to samsara.

Another way to remember it is to bring the mala to the level of the heart, to underline the devotional aspect of the practice and the intentional effort to transcend the lower levels of being.

The use of mala gives the body an action to perform, helping it to let restlessness go. The Mantra is repeated with each pearl, making them slide between thumb and middle finger. With use, pearls are spiritualized.

How to Get the Best Benefits by Using a Mantra

To get more benefits from your mantra practice you can follow these simple recommendations which represent the ideal situation for any spiritual practice:

- Try to practice as much as possible, but remember that in any case, if you practice with concentration and devotion, you will always get great benefits.
- It is good to establish a period of time for daily practice and continue at least until you begin to experience its effects. A good start is to practice for at least three months.

- The most recommended time is very early in the morning (around four). If you cannot practice in that time, you can still do it at another time that is more compatible with your lifestyle. It would be good to at least be able to practice at the same time at least, because it helps you to maintain regularity in the practice and to let your day be marked by spiritual practice.

- It is better to wait at least an hour and a half after eating food.

- Before starting, it is a good habit to take a bath or at least wash your hands, face and feet. While washing, one can visualize washing the impurities of the mind. By wearing clean clothes, we visualize the soul that takes on its divine nature.

- Choose a calm place, facing north or east. We delimit our sacred space with wool or pure silk, in order to conserve energy and keep away the most material vibrations. For the same reason, a shawl of natural fibers is used to cover the body, which also helps to preserve the spiritual vibrations produced during the practice.

- The vertebral column must be straight, so that the current of prana (life force) which is created and stimulated by song can flow freely. This pranic circuit should be closed by sitting cross-legged.

- Your hands rest on your lap, with your palms facing upward to suggest abandonment and receptivity. You should try to be as relaxed as possible in the position. Find out more about yogic relaxation.
- The gaze must be concentrated in the space between the eyebrows.
- At the beginning and end of the practice, you can offer a thank you prayer to everyone who sang the Mantra. After practice, sit on your quiet, receptive mat in a natural state of silent meditation. Exit the practice gently and slowly, trying to keep peace as long as possible.
- If you can, avoid starting another business immediately.

The mind may need a concrete image to stay focused during Mantra practice. In Bhakti yoga, the yoga of love and devotion, the devotee focuses on the image of the divinity connected to the Mantra (the Ishta Devata). We can use an image that we have painted ourselves, take it from a book or use the photograph of our spiritual Master.

Chapter 4: Yantras And Mandalas

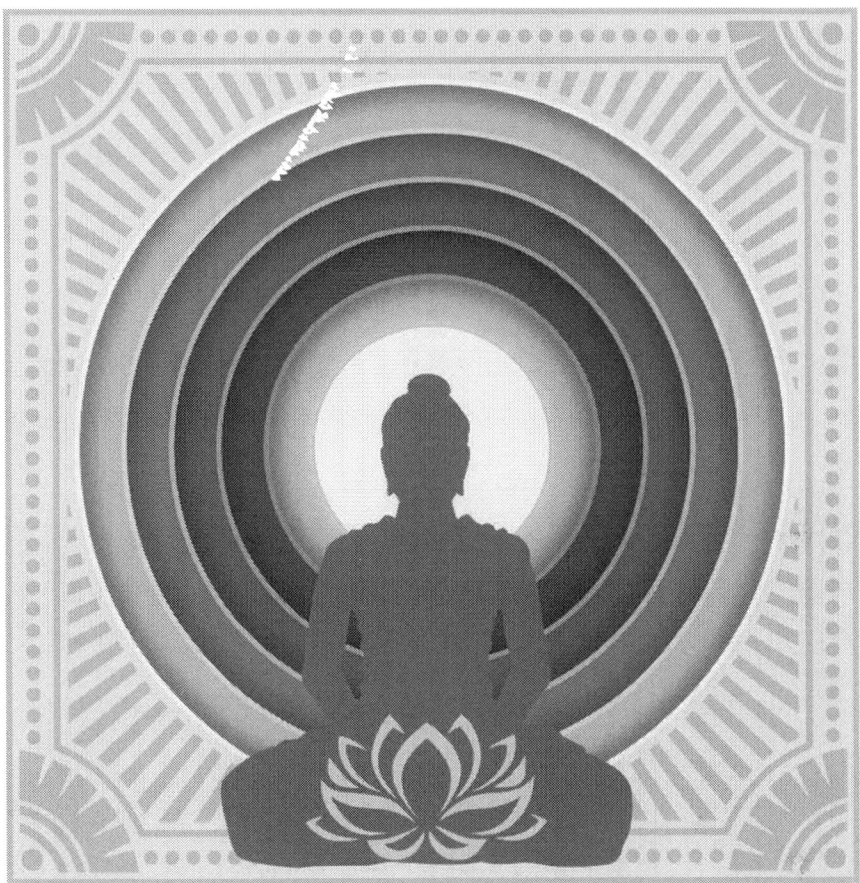

Yantra are powerful visual tools for meditation, their origin and use are reminiscent of those of the mandalas, they represent symbolic compositions of the vibratory sequences of a particular divinity. Unlike the mantras which are the mind, consciousness, spirit and name of the divinity (devata) the yantra is its body. This is how ancient tantric researchers perceived it in their vision. In this regard the Kularnav Tantra says:

"Yantram Mantram Mayam Proktam
Mantatim Devataiv Hi
Dehat Manor Yathe Bhedo
Tantra Devatayostatha. "

The meaning is that divinity pervades mantra and yantra in the same way, different from each other as mind and body. When a yantra is the object of worship and its energy is invoked, it is transformed into the symbolic representation of the divinity that manifests itself only when the critical and analytical state of mind is overlooked, and then the energy flows to the higher centers.

Each yantra becomes the residence of the divinity whose name it bears. The essence of divinity is in the iconography of the yantra that represents it and there will never be such powerful idols or images.

An idol is a personal representation, while the Yantra which is made of archetypal forms common to every existing phenomenology, is universal. Hence, a yantra is an archetypal unit, even in the process of a constructive realization phase, a process that takes us from a concrete reality to an abstract one.

In Sanskrit yantra means machine or instrument, it comes from the root yam which means support, contain, maintain and from the syllable trana "liberation". If the expression becomes symbolic it becomes yam as yama the lord of death, between "accessing" and trana "freedom", then a yantra "free from death" (cycle of death and rebirth) giving moksha (liberation). But the main definition of mantra is that it contains the energies of the divinity it symbolizes. The symbols are precise and unchanging ways of expression which, in essence, correspond to the inner life, intense and qualitative as it is everlasting and qualitative is eternal life. In the symbol, the detail represents the general, and is a creative representation of the irreversible. This makes the Yantra a reflection of the divine. When the yantra is understood as a symbol, it becomes every symbol and every symbol is a yantra.

As a tool, the yantra is used to withdraw consciousness from the external world and situate it in the internal one, helping the sadhaka (practitioner) to go beyond the ordinary register of the mind, towards an altered state of consciousness (turiya).

How is a Yantra made

Usually the yantra consists of a square frame in which triangles, lotus petals, circles are inscribed. Structurally the yantra consists exclusively of geometric figures; instead, figures, places and objects of complex and meticulous execution appear in the mandala.

As for meaning, the mandala represents the physical and psychic universe, the yantra a particular divinity or cosmic force. The mandala is mainly used in the Buddhist context, the yantra in the Hindu one, and the symbols that compose it are derived from Tantrism, Hindu esotericism.

Below some of the most important symbols that constitute a yantra and their significance:

- the central point is the origin of the universe, space and time; it also represents the unity of the female and male poles; It is also called Bindu: it symbolizes the essence of the universe, the absolute principle from which the creation, the union between the Male and the Female, arose; at the same time it brings back to the center of one's self putting in harmony and vibration both the divine and the human consciousness inserted and enveloped in the composition.

- the circle represents universal Consciousness, which expands from the One (the central point) and then divides itself to create the whole manifest world;
- the triangle, facing downwards, is connected to the female energy (Shakti, companion of Shiva); facing upwards it represents the male principle (Shiva)
- the square is the symbol of the Earth element;
- the lotus flower, represents the Sun or the Moon (according to the number of petals), is the only non-geometric element and symbolizes the pure mind of those who meditate seeking enlightenment.

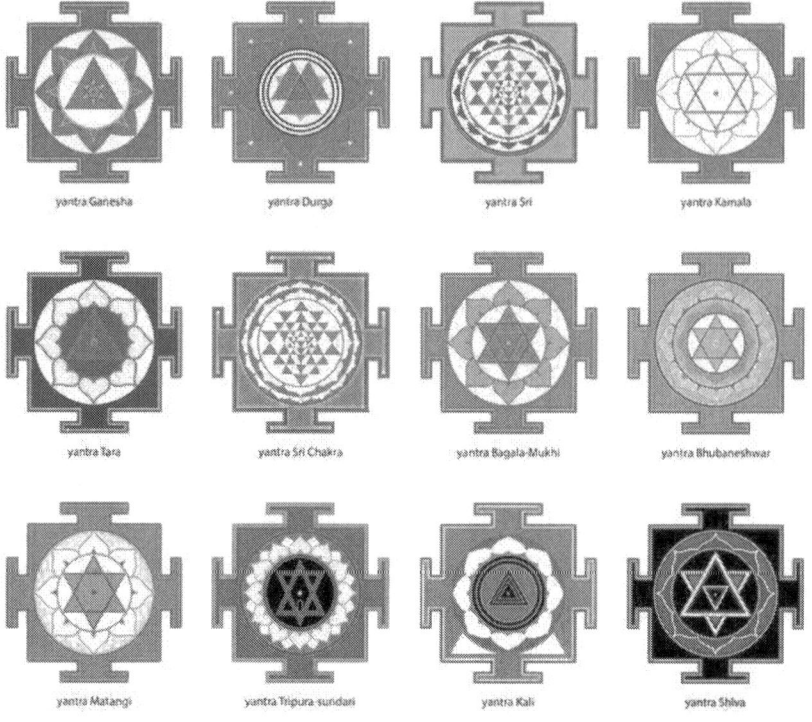

Yantras

The mandala can be considered to represent a cosmogram, an illustration of the universe, and the yantra a "theogram", an illustration of the divine. But the real function of both is to evoke the energetic aspect of the cosmos or divinity, and above all to open up to other states of consciousness, extra-ordinary, to learn to read in the human tissue (the microcosm) the plots of the universe (the macrocosm).

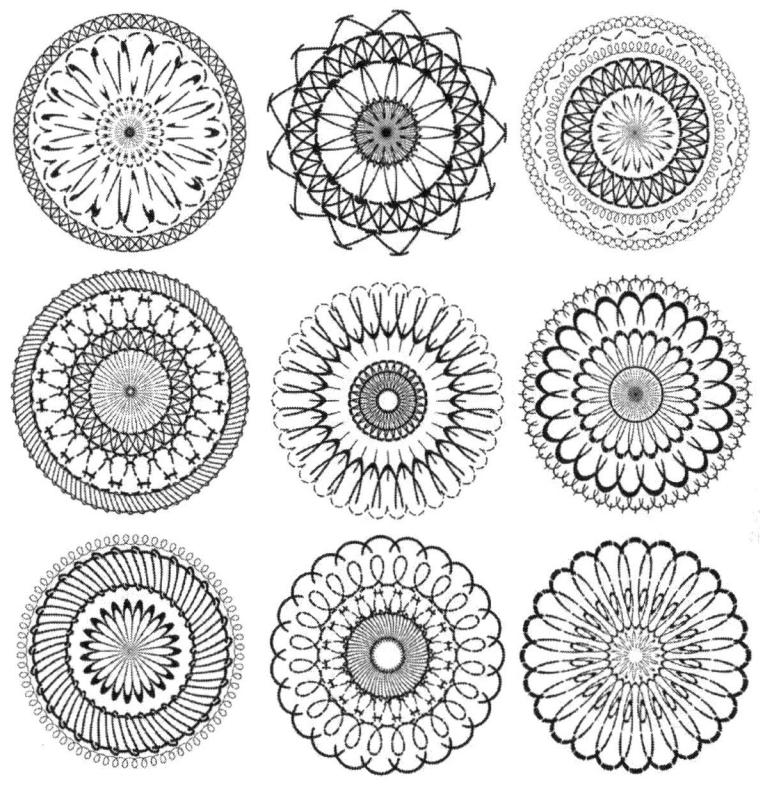

Mandalas

Designed on fabric, on a leaf, on paper, on wood, or even engraved on stone or metal, the yantra is a geometric representation, painted with various colors, and represents a divinity (evoked with appropriate formulas - mantra - and considered present in the drawing during the cults), indeed it is the body itself. Indian women draw yantra at the entrance door to keep away bad energies; Yantras are also present in Hindu sanctuaries to represent the Universe and evoke one of the thousand deities of the Hindu pantheon. In Vastu, the "yoga of living" (a sort of ancient Indian version of Feng Shui), the yantra are used to place the right energies inside the house.

The use of yantra is one of the fundamental parts of the tantric rite, that is of that specific religious system composed of rituals and practices that is based on Tantra, a series of doctrinal texts. According to this vision, the adept can achieve spiritual progress thanks also to the proper use of yantra (together with a whole series of other practices including yoga, mudras, mantras ...): the devotee, in fact, meditating on them, can evoke the energy of the divinity represented by the geometric diagram. Among other things, they are also appreciated at the most popular level and also have an apotropaic and protection from evil function. The yantra are, so to speak, the visual equivalent of mantras and are considered, as previously anticipated, powerful designs that with an appropriate rite make you "alive". Parent of the most famous mandalas (from which, however, they are distinguished by some characteristics), the yantra may seem to be only geometrical and dry designs: in reality, as we have seen, they enclose a symbolic universe and religious of great suggestion and charm.

Mandala how it works

The "drawings" symbols of the beauty of the universe and the microcosm of Man allow you to concentrate on obtaining a new awareness, which helps you to be closer to what the symbol represents.

For example, if you are looking for harmony in your life, you can help yourself by drawing and / or coloring the corresponding mandala. Choosing where to tattoo a mandala is not a random choice. Shoulders, arms and legs are the best places to protect yourself or to face a difficulty in life. The mandala can be read from the outside to the inside.

The word "Mandala" is in Sanskrit. In a circle that delimits a space, different geometric figures (= point, triangle and square) are inserted to focus on what you are looking for in life. This differentiates the mandala from the yantra, which instead represents advice and warnings.

In the West, the symbol was used to represent Christ, from which four points were derived (= the Evangelists). In the eastern world, however, the symbol is a spiritual journey, which allows you to get closer to your own nature and to what surrounds us.

Let's see how to read a mandala. It starts from the circle, which represents consciousness and the cycle of life. The square, on the other hand, indicates rationality. The point is the beginning or origin of the whole. Finally, the triangle is the direction to follow.

In addition to these symbols, there is the cross, the link between the earthly and spiritual world; and the spiral, which unites the psyche and creativity.

Numbers and colors have their own particular meaning. Numbers have these meanings:

- The individual.
- The opposites.
- The harmony.
- Balance and strength.
- Physicality.
- The creativity.
- Completion of a stage in life.

Here is the meaning of the different colors:

- Black is the pain
- White is the change

- Vitality is red
- Orange is the will to succeed
- Yellow is awareness
- Blue is motherhood
- Viola is creativity

Ganesha Yantra mandala

The elephant-headed god Ganesh removes obstacles, and the Ganesha yantra brings good luck and success to new ventures. Just as the elephant moves in the jungle, slowly but surely, sweeping away the leaves and branches in front of it, the god Ganesh helps to eliminate obstacles.

If we perceive the existence of "blocks" in our life, and / or we need direction, creativity and abundance, we can meditate on this yantra. However, the yogi can make use of the yantra only when he has reached a certain level in his spiritual progress, since using them involves many preliminary acts: evoking the divinity within himself, transferring it to the yantra through a ritual of consecration and accompanying it with the recitation of appropriate mantras and the execution of appropriate mudras (symbolic gestures).

Chapter 5: Tantric Meditation

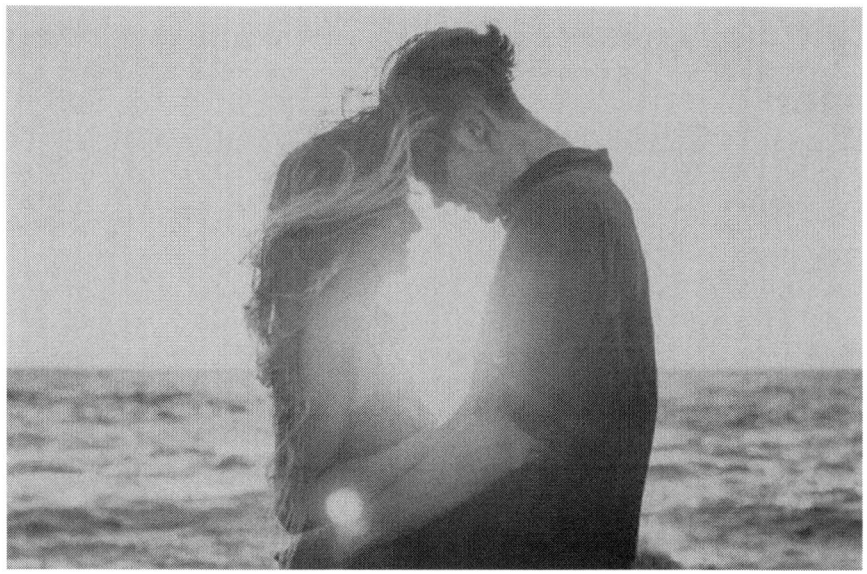

Tantric meditation is an active and fundamental part of tantric thought, at the center of which is the manifest of universe, created as a physical and sensorial expression of the un-manifest. It is through immersion in the former that full unity with the latter becomes possible. This however entails a rigid discipline, variable according to the practitioner's level of consciousness. However, each level has as its common denominator the work on the harmonization of male and female energy, Shiva and Shakty, which are also close to the Taoist concepts of Yin and Yang. The aim of this activity is to properly awaken and channel Kundalini energy, the custodian of the secret of enlightenment. Tantric philosophy has roots both in archaic Buddhism and Hinduism, but it is believed that Hinduism inherited the tantra from Buddhism, and not vice versa, since the oldest Tantra (philosophical reference texts) are of Buddhist compilation and date back to 350 AD. Today, tantric meditation and more generally tantrism are known in the chronicles as techniques to improve sexual performance or to intervene in difficult situations as a couple. Most of what is said about it is limiting, if not completely wrong.

Basic tantric meditation helps the practitioner to find peace and balance, as it manages to connect each phase which, during everyday life, remains disconnected from the others. Integration occurs because, during tantra practice, emotions and different attitudes are combined together, with harmony. In addition to this, given the structuring and repetitiveness of tantra practice, this type of meditation can be effective as a stabilizing factor in a society that is characterized by being destabilizing. Meditation thus helps to make life flow in an interrupted flow of continuity. With regard to the sexual dimension of the practice, the tantric approach helps to alleviate the couple's tensions, bringing benefits in case of frigidity, premature ejaculation and even impotence, when this has psychological roots.

Methods of Tantric mediation

The different teachings of the masters, which have followed one another over the centuries, use very similar techniques, having a solid common basis. The extinction of the samskaras, the accumulated karmic seeds that prevent the expansion of consciousness. An example of meditative process that is based on Tantric tradition is the one proposed below:

- Iiswara Pranidhana: the practitioner, through different stages, develops awareness of his own deep spiritual nature. In this first stage, the conditionings of the mind and the karma of past lives are slowly removed

- Madhu vidya: the practitioner introduces meditation into daily life

- Tattva dharana: through the use of meditative tools, such as mantra and yantra, the practitioner begins the deep purification of the subtle elements, dissolving the nodes in the nadis (channels through which, in traditional Indian medicine and spiritual knowledge, the energies such as prana of the physical body, the subtle body and the causal body are said to flow) and raising the level of the kundalini

- Pranayama: through a breathing technique typical of yoga, the yogi controls his own vital energy, placing it at the service of the development of consciousness

- Shodana: a system of deep purification and empowerment of the potentials of the subtle centers of the body is developed
- Dhyana: this phase of meditation leads the practitioner to abandon the meditative supports used to merge with his half.

You can also start meditating with simpler techniques, which can be learned during a course that is not limited to asanas only.

Tantric or tantra meditation can also be used in a couple's relationship, not necessarily with therapeutic intent, but also as a way of knowing the other. Unlike what can be expected, tantra is not a guide to sex, but a spiritual path that can also be done in a couple whose goal is awareness. There is no precise starting point, a precise arrival point is not described, but paths are identified that do not necessarily have to do with sexual intercourse, which aim to unlock the energies. Men and women are carriers of complementary and different energy flows that can "blossom" thanks to common meditation. These techniques can be used by sexologists to improve the couple's affinity and knowledge before tackling any problems immediately on a physical level.

Mantra meditation

For "formal" meditation with mantras, adopt a sitting posture. For casual practice, you can repeat the mantra in the back of your mind, with your eyes open, during other daily doings.

Singing the mantra energizes you quickly. Scanning it with a certain cadence calms the mind. If your repetition is too fast or too slow, it will become an automatic process and your mind will wander too much or fall prey to sleep.

The rapidity with which the mantra is spelled out also varies according to the length of the mantra: short ones (from one to three syllables) are often reiterated more slowly than long mantras.

Since the speed varies according to the technique you are adopting, the advise is to experiment with different repetition speeds and find out which one is the most effective. It is better to maintain a uniform repetition rate rather than changing it several times during a practice.

If your mind is very active and full of thoughts, it may be useful to "increase the volume" in repeating the mantra, making it stronger and more incisive. If, on the other hand, your mind is quieter, the mantra can become more subtle and be recited in a low voice, like a high-frequency sound that can barely be heard. The word itself is almost gone and the mantra is perceived more as sound vibrations than as a punctuated phrase.

You may or may not be capable to synch the mantra with your breath. Some options to do it better are:

- Inhale and exhale as you say the mantra. If the mantra is very small, like om, you can repeat it one time while inhaling, and one more while exhaling. You can also increase your speed and repeat it three times for each inhalation and three times for exhalation. If the mantra is lengthy, then you can recite half of it during inspiration and the second half while exhaling.
- Exhale. Inhale without reciting the mantra, and spell out the mantra only on exhalation.

Just focus on the mantra, paying attention to breathing. With time, the breath tends to synchronize naturally with the rhythm of the mantra.

Progressing on Mantra meditation

The more we reiterate our mantra, the more we give it energy. A one-syllable mantra, it is thought that after 125,000 reiterations "gets its own life". It is our repetitive attention that works with the mantra and loads it. The mantra then gets to be the strongest thought in your mind, and then you can really count on it to give you peace and concentration into your life.

Once the mantra gets this momentum, repetition becomes easier. It is as if once we manage to "start" or "access" the mantra then it goes on by itself, bringing us into a state of internal silence.

The following is the typical progress of the practice:

- Verbal acting - repeat it aloud. This simple mechanism involves your senses, facilitating in keeping your attention focused.
- The whisper: the mouths and the tongue move, but only produce a faint sound. This part is more subtle and profound than verbal acting.
- Mental recitation - reiterate the mantra only in your mind. At the beginning, of course, there will be some action in the tongue and throat, but over time they too

will stop, and the exercise will be entirely in the mind. This stage is the most common in mantra meditation.

- Spontaneous listening - at this stage you are no longer reiterating the mantra, but the mantra continues naturally alone in your mind. No need to worry about the intensity and speed. Just pay attention to the Mantra repeating it as it naturally wants to be reiterated. This stage is referred as ajapa japa.

There is a slow but significant progression from the first to the last level. A very common mistake in beginners is to want to skip stages and go directly to the mental stage, or spontaneous repetition. Although it is not impossible to get there immediately, it is much easier to follow this scale to master meditation with mantras.

Even if you dislike verbal acting and want to jump straight to the mental level, I recommend that you do at least a few cycles of acting whispered at the beginning. This will help you focus your brain on the mantra.

Wherever you are on this progression, if you find out that your mind is disengaging from the mantra, distracted by other thoughts or sleepy, stop for a few seconds and then employ a more conscious action in repeating the mantra, until you come to an effective result.

Yantra meditation

As explained earlier, Yantras are geometric designs conceived as containers of spiritual energies. In the Himalayan region of northern India, where traces of their use were found in 2000 BC, they are still used today to cultivate the universal properties of devotion and purification, for the spirit. The practice originates from the "mantras" (vibration of sounds) and the yantra are the visual representation of the vibrations, and are part of the philosophical practice of Tantra.

If you are interested in deepening meditation, but you are not comfortable with the traditional method of sitting in silence, or you want to experiment with a different technique, the creation of yantra can be for you. The yantra images are the symbol of your personal research. Studying the trait, the shape, the color, becoming aware of the time and the devotion that the realization requires, are the ingredients for realizing the inner beauty. You will be surprised by the power of the creative force that emanates. The power of work through the use of these symbols continues to manifest itself even after unconsciously creation within you. The yantra can be taken with you, at home, in the office and remain a foothold for a calm and positive energy recharge. Specific effects of the practice depend on the type of design you choose to work with.

Now you can choose a shape or shapes which to some extent are in greater resonance with you. Or even better, redesign them by comparing yourself with the process, patience, observation and attention required. Or make a color copy and internalize it by meditating on it. If you intend to color it, use pastels, start from the top and continue clockwise, from the outside until you get to the bindu, the point in the center. Working in this direction, you visualize the internalization process, which symbolically proceeds "from the outside of the chatter of the mind" towards a spiral movement that takes you inside the immutable part of the self. Each color has been chosen to emit frequencies that resonate within the shape, so it is advisable to stay within the chosen color scheme. For example the passion yantra must always be red, but feel free to choose the red tone you like best. Coloring is an important part of the meditation process, live it with awareness.

Choose your Yantra

Before starting meditation, choose your yantra.

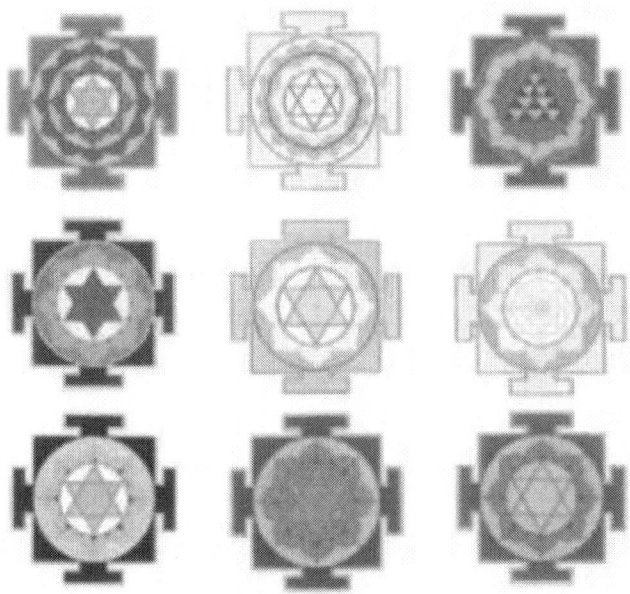

Let your eyes run on these 9 diagrams and focus on what attracts you most. Do not read the box (the 9 qualities) on the following page. Allow the shapes and colors to speak to you instinctively. Observe the qualities that the instinctive choice of yantra has shown you.

Redesign it, color it and listen to the feeling that evokes you.

Meaning of the Yantras

First column on the left

- high: radiance. sunshine, optimism, self-confidence, magnetism. It allows your joy, warmth and energy to influence those you interact with.
- middle: intellect. judgment, balance, wisdom. calms the nervous system and invites the mind to an equanimous attitude.
- Low: organization. order, discipline, steady mind. Patience and endurance are rooted.

Column in the Center

- high: nourishment. Protection, sustenance, compassion. cultivates the qualities of openness, sensitivity and transformation typically associated with women.
- middle: expansion. growth, opulence, luck, generosity of spirit, community creation. opens the heart to opportunities, to sharing and to new horizons.
- low: uniqueness. independence, originality, exploration. Awareness of one's ideas and knowledge of "one's own true voice".

Column on the Right

- high: Passion. direction, goals, enthusiasm. It allows you to live your aspirations and goals with joy and richness of meaning.

- middle: bliss. sensuality, admiration for beauty, re-finement, art. opens access to the joyful aspects of the senses.
- low: spirituality. Mystical experience, loneliness, purifi-cation. the wisdom that always lives with you.

Start the Meditation

After choosing your Yantra, get in a comfortable position. The bindu (center of the yantra) is the focal point on which you must pay attention; so put it at a height, on the ground or on a table, where the gaze does not struggle to observe it. Gently stare at the center of your yantra for a few minutes: you will see the colors and shapes around in peripheral vision widen. Retrace the path of choice, design, shape and coloring. After fixing it intensely, close your eyes and internalize the shape with the mind's eye. As you watch the contours and colors slowly fade, pay attention to the feelings of tranquility that grow in you. The steps and paths for weaving (Tantra) of this practice may change depending on the type of diagram chosen, but ultimately they all lead to the same place, the quiet truth.

Benefits of tantric meditation to improve sexual life

Limits stress – Tantric Meditation manages to regulate the production of chemicals by the brain, increasing the levels of serotonin and dopamine and decreasing those of cortisol and adrenaline, related to stress. The reason is very simple: the mind is kept focused on physical breathing and not on anxiety. In so doing, the body relaxes and is more prone to sex. Indeed, women would be unable to orgasm due to fatigue and stress.

Makes you more empathetic - Empathy is the ability to understand a person's mood, feeling emotional participation in everything that happens to him/her. Thanks to meditation, this quality would be stimulated because the so-called "mirror neurons" of the brain would be activated, that is, the main responsible for the ability to intuit the feelings that people are feeling. In sexual intercourse, therefore, one no longer concentrates solely on oneself but focuses on the moment itself.

Intimacy increases - With meditation you feel more focused and spiritual, as if you are more connected to what you live. The muscles, therefore, become elastic, articulated, fluid, soft and the mind becomes free, allowing you to find greater intimacy with your partner. In this way, sex becomes a real sensory experience.

Who is it suitable for?

Tantric meditation is a practice open to all, both for those who prefer to be alone and for those who intend to involve a partner in their spiritual journey. In the latter case, it will be possible to grow with the other half of the couple, meditating in sexual union or experimenting with other techniques to expand awareness. Tantrism allows you to have both a partner in the form displayed and a true partner, in both cases, you will achieve the same results since your meditative state will not be influenced by the real presence of a person. A similar activity is especially recommended for those who feel stressed, tired and exhausted due to the frenzy of daily life since it allows you to find harmony with the surrounding world and enjoy life minute by minute. Tantric meditation has not only beneficial effects on the psyche but also on the body. The exercises practiced strengthen the pubococcygeus muscles, reducing the likelihood of prostate problems in men, while in women they help tone the hormonal system, avoiding hormone-dependent osteoporosis.

Chapter 6: Shiva And Shakti, Yin And Yang

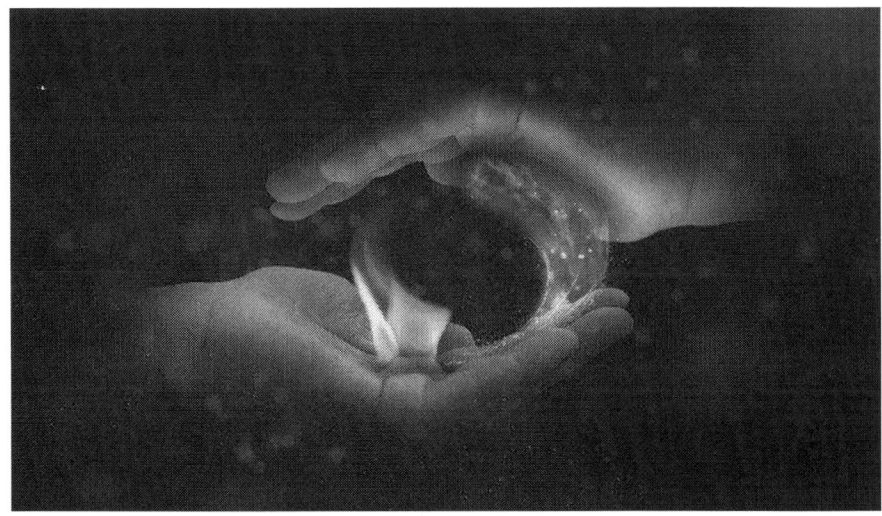

Much is said today about tantric practices of domination of sexual energy (although tantra is mostly a model of thought and does not necessarily refer to sex), but not everyone knows that there are two main tantric traditions, the first is that Indian and the second is the Taoist one. Sexuality is what allows a spiritual soul to reach the dimensions of form and gravitation, but since the entrance door can also be the exit door, if used appropriately it gives the human being the possibility to detach himself from the weight of the gravitation and approaching the upper thin dimensions.

According to the Tantric vision, creation is not a process that began at a defined or definable moment in time, the same applies to dissolution / death, in fact both processes take place and have always followed each other since ever: what exists and happens now, outside and inside ourselves, is perfectly analogous to what happened to the "origins". This continuous process can be defined in one word: Evolution which is the purpose and identity of the Creation / Dissolution process.

Sex as sacred energy

Many ancient traditions, western and eastern, considered sex the sacred energy par excellence. In particular, Tantra as one of the highest spiritual ways from ancient origins. The consideration that unified these traditions was that everything in the universe comes from sexual energy, from conjunction and fusion of polar opposites.

In India, Tibet and China this united vision reaches its apogee: the divinities are represented together and often in the position of the loving act. It should be noted that in Tantra as in the other spiritual ways, the sexual position is almost never lying down, but sitting, so as to make it vertical the inner psychophysical axis. This allows you to experience the loving act as meditation, transforming it from animal instinct into spiritual and evolutionary practice.

In ancient India Tantrism adored the two poles of existence: Shiva, the male God, who is symbolically depicted with a lingam, an erect phallus of stone, marble, ice (as ad Amarnath) or metal, while Shakti, his consort, with a yoni, of oval or circular shape. It is common to find these in various temples two united and interpenetrated symbols that are venerated as an image same as the divine. Shiva and Shakti are the archetypes of consciousness and energy.

In Tantra sexual union is the foundation of the structure metaphysics itself: the entire universe arises from sexual union of immaterial consciousness with creative energy. In every physical atom (well known to Indians), in every living thing vegetable or animal, as in every star in the cosmos, the type energy material hides and implies an inner consciousness. There is no matter-energy without its aspect of consciousness immanent.

The sexual relationship, which is at the origin of the whole existence, explains how every new life, every form comes from a sexual act. The pulse and rhythm of the love act can be found in every aspect of life in the form of a cycle, vibration or pulsation, from the planets, to the seasons, to the beat of the heart and breath. All existence is perceived as a continuous creative act that arises from the incessant love relationship of consciousness and energy.

This tantric, unitary and evolutionary vision is transmitted from India to Tibet and China where it takes on the symbol of Tao in which the two polar forces Yin and Yang balance. The Taoist vision is absolutely parallel to the tantric one, both for the awareness that the essence of consciousness is present in every manifestation of existence and for the understanding that all stems from the balance of the female and the male. It is interesting to remember that Niels Bohr, the great physicist of Copenhagen school, used the Tao symbol as
element of understanding the quantum mystery of existence.

The Indian tradition – Shiva and Shakti

Everything that exists is manifested by the continuous interaction between two opposite poles: one essentially static - Shiva (which however also has dynamic aspects), and the other essentially dynamic - Shakti (which also presents static aspects). The external part of each shape and each phenomenon represents the fruit of the creative aspect of a dynamic force, in the internal part there is a static force which constitutes the core of creation, the heart of phenomenal existence.

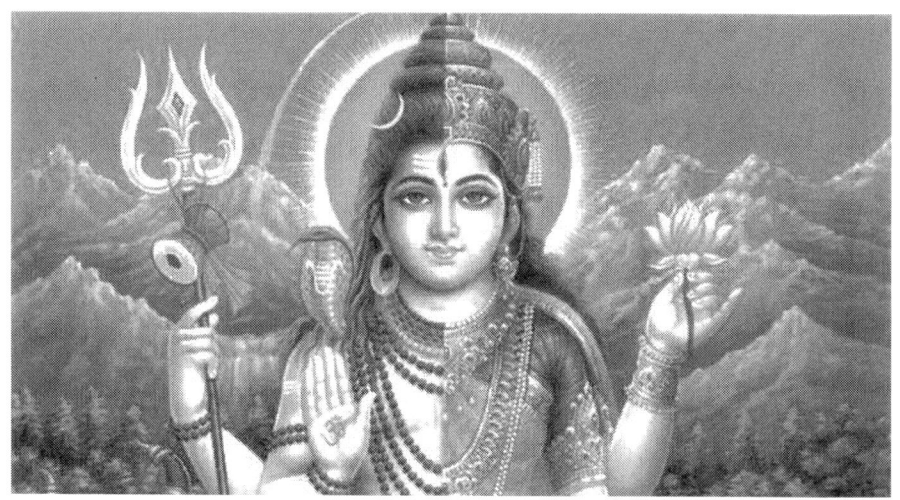

The SHIVA PURANA states that "the whole universe was created by SHIVA and SHAKTI". They symbolize two opposite polarities, two absolute and eternal principles: the Male and the Female, which through their union give life to the whole manifestation.

The Hindu Pantheon is populated with divinities; almost all have a counterpart, since each higher principle is believed to exist only through a combination of masculine and feminine. Consequently, each male divinity is conceived as inseparable from a female contrary Energy or SHAKTI.

The term Tantra comes from Sanskrit and means "weft and warp" (and also "method"), it indicates a series of ancient sacred texts of an esoteric and magical nature and in full the discipline that derives from those teachings (developed in India around to the IV-V century AD).

Tantric doctrine foresees the identity between matter and spirit, individual soul (jivatman) and universal soul (paramatman), the latter foundation of all things, indivisible, transcendent and eternal. The manifestation comes from the dynamic interaction of the male creative principle (purusha) and primordial energy-matter (prakriti), identified with the divinities of Shiva and Shakti and symbolized by the lingam (phallus) and the yoni (vagina). The reunification of the two sexes eliminates the polarity of opposites and leads back to the original indivisible Unity, through the overcoming of existential dualism.

Tantric rites have strong magical-symbolic connotations and involve the use of mudras (particular positions of the hands and fingers), bija and mantra (verbal recitations composed - respectively - by one or more syllables), mandalas (circular diagrams that symbolically represent the created universe) and yantra (geometric diagrams composed of lines, triangles and concentric circles that represent the convergence of the multiple in unity).

Through the act of sexual reunion the union of Shiva with Shakti is celebrated until it reaches the complete dominion of cosmic energies. Unlike the purely contemplative ways, which preached estrangement from the world, Tantrism introduced the concept of participating in the game of existence (including sexual play) without identifying yourselves, rather by using poison (passion and appetite for the senses) that obscure the true understanding of Reality) as a remedy, and it is true that in times of darkness like the present one (kali yuga) tantra is perhaps one of the few methods that can lead us back to Unity. However, even in tantrism there are purist contemplative currents, in which sexual union is not foreseen (they are the Paths of the right hand) and in which the initiate reaches the union between Shiva and Shakti only within himself, in the rites - on the other hand - in which the participation of the woman is foreseen, we speak of the "Way of the left hand".

In Indian tantric practice, devotion, prayer to the divine Mother, the spiritual idealization of the partner, which for the woman becomes a representation of the Lord Shiva (whose symbol in the yantra is a higher vertex triangle) is fundamental. Man of Divine Shakti (triangle with lower vertex). The participants in the act of sacred union must be able to visualize themselves as divinities: man must meditate on himself in the role of Shiva, Lord of Transcendence, maintaining the balance of energies with the control of breath, thought and seed, and the woman must visualize herself as a pure expression of the primordial Shakti, embodiment of the power of eros.

The role of Shiva

"SHIVA is Pure Existence, the immortal Divine Principle. SHIVA is pure Consciousness, unconditional and transcendent. SHIVA is the divinity of the mind, the Lord of Yoga, the Master of the three worlds and the winner over death." (SHIVA PURANA)

SHIVA is the principle of the centrifugal force by means of which every life, every shape, every cosmic system dissolves in the infinite immensity of the divine. Everything originates in him. He is the expanding force of the world, he is the energy source of existence, the principle of life, but also the principle of dissolution and transformation.

The transcendental force of SHIVA is a gateway that leads beyond earthly things; it goes from the mundane to the metaphysical and gives birth to an understanding of the real nature of existence. It is the penetrating power of pure undifferentiated consciousness; is the ecstatic transcendent quality of evolution. Heaven and earth find their synthesis in SHIVA, since He is also in the world, in nature, in animals, in the very thirst for life of every living being.

SHIVA means "Benign" and from this point of view it constitutes the beneficial aspect of divinity, while the terrible aspect is represented by RUDRA or "Flaming", the one who makes tears flow.

Positive / negative dualism always characterizes the figure of SHIVA. These are apparently contradictory components but in reality they refer to different aspects in which divinity manifests itself. In fact, his hypostases are numerous (1008) and each expresses some specific characteristics that are specific to him.

Since everything pulsates, everything has a frequency; SHIVA is also the Lord of rhythm and dance and as such gives growth to the creation of shapes. His most important and well-known artistic representation is NATARAJA, SHIVA the Lord of Dance. Dance, thought a type of mysticism as it enables to free the supernatural powers of the danseur, characterizes a real creative action in SHIVA.

As we have already mentioned, SHIVA cannot be conceived without its female half, the SHAKTI. He can only become active when the energy of the SHAKTI gives him strength. Without SHAKTI, SHIVA becomes SHAVA, that is, a lifeless body.

The role of Shakti

SHAKTI: from the root "shak" means being able to do, to have the strength to do, to act; basically it means power. It is the universal rule of vitality, strength and creativeness. SHAKTI is inseparable from the one who owns her - SHAKTIMAN, male principle or Universal Father. The universe is the product of this pair of opposites: one static (SHAKTIMAN) the other dynamic (SHAKTI). The external part of everything is the creative aspect of dynamic force, and within each dynamic creature there is static a force, which is the core of phenomenal existence.

SHIVA and SHAKTI create the antagonism of the basic principles of the universe; the number one is the spirit, the cosmic man (PURUSHA), the number two is the energy of the world (PRAKRITI). The whole manifestation is the product of energy that derives from the power of their union that generates bliss; that is, it is the product of joy and pleasure.

The conjunction of SHIVA and SHAKTI symbolizes the impulse to bring together "being", awareness and power, energy, transcendent aspect and immanent aspect. SHIVA is precisely being, immutability, the nature of the atma or conscious principle; in SHAKTI it is precisely movement, change; it is the origin of all production, generation and vivification.

SHAKTI represents the strength not yet implemented in the shape of SHIVA; SHIVA is that which is united and transformed in it, reunified with itself, transparent and luminous. In particular, the first corresponds to everything that is matter, body and mind, the second the conscious principle; both therefore present themselves in Tantrism only as two ways of viewing of a single principle, of a single reality. Their supreme synthesis is comparable to a flame that has consumed all matter and is now only itself, as pure energy or pure act.

It is known that to help the universe and all its beings, SHIVA, as a total neutral, split into two harmonizing entities. From the union of God and Goddess every living reality is formed. From the union of the mystical couple, the whole universe proceeds in both its static and stable and dynamic aspects; both in intangible and conscious forms, and in intangible and unconscious ones. The active / passive, male / female elements, which appear only in their opposition, are in truth only one. In Hindu iconography this thought is represented by an androgynous figure, half male and half female, which synthetically contains all the aspects and characteristics of the two polarities: ARDHANARISHVARA.

The union of Shiva and Shakti

Although most spiritual traditions consider sexuality as something "dirty" and "low", according to Tantra erotic energy can be used to explore parts of themselves that are still unknown, improve the connection you have with the partner and open up to a deeper understanding of love and understanding of the universe around us.

Sex in fact, according to the tantric tradition, is sacred and symbolizes the union between Shiva and Shakti: Shiva the embodiment of the male principle, static, aware, conscious, Shakti the embodiment of the female principle, energetic, vital and in constant change.

According to the tantric vision, the ever changing dance of Shakti around Shiva, the immovable witness and central axis of the dance, is what creates and maintains the universe.

Shiva and Shakti in sexual rituals

During tantric sexual rituals the two lovers recreate this reunion through the mystical union, in which they become two divinities themselves thanks to a process of mutual transfiguration, internally realizing the perfect Androginal State.

During the love act with consecration, continence and transfiguration, man and woman embody the two divine principles, SHIVA and SHAKTI, which merge into a cosmic embrace intoxicating with infinite bliss. The human couple becomes a Divine, Cosmic Couple and transforms a physical act into a sacred moment in which sublime, elevated, ecstatic inner experiences are produced which lead to higher states of consciousness and allow the realization of the Absolute.

The transfiguration process of course must not remain limited to the ambit of love fusion. At all times, two beings who love each other must transfigure themselves and the other as SHAKTI or SHIVA. Man must recognize in woman the embodiment of SHAKTI, the manifestation of primordial creative energy, and worship her as a Goddess, just as woman must recognize in man the embodiment of SHIVA, the manifestation of Divine Consciousness and express in his devotion and infinite love.

Each woman, identifying with SHAKTI will assimilate its specific attributes. It will begin to manifest a splendid, irresistible energy that it expresses through passion, but also a profound beauty, delicacy, inner grace and harmony. It will demonstrate wisdom, compassion and calm, but also strength, power and an iron will.

An authentic SHAKTI exudes the spell of sweetness that intoxicates its SHIVA with divine; he is capable of transmitting profound happiness and transforming life into a wonderful bliss. With its enchanting power, existence becomes a celestial work, which reveals the mystical secrets of ecstasy and which reveals the rhythm of the harmonies of the power of creation.

Yin and Yang in the Taoist tradition

According to the basic tantric principles, sex is used to combine female energy and male energy and create, through the union of two poles, an explosion that leads both practitioners to transcend the manifestation. This is obviously the ultimate goal, but there are also intermediate goals such as opening oneself up to love, improving complicity with the partner, intimately feeling the other as if he were himself.

To create the "critical mass" that allows practitioners to open to the Infinite (or at least part of it), it is essential that the two parts are "polarized", one of Yang energy ("male") and the other of Yin ("female") energy. Polarizing energy, in the specific case of sex, means that

- For the bearer of male (Yang), energy must take on maximum masculine attributes, that is, pure awareness, pure consciousness, immovability and constancy
- For the bearer of female (Yin) energy must take full advantage of female attributes, such as vitality, sensitivity to emotions, attitude to change.

For this reason, in Tantra, at least in the use of sensuality as a tool to transcend, women are trying to become more "feminine" and men more "masculine". In Tantra it has been observed that generally the male body is mainly charged with Yang energy and the female body is generally charged with Ying energy.

In Taoism the universe is represented as a natural opposition and dynamic game of yin energy (cold, descending, female) and yang energy (hot, ascending, male), we speak - albeit a little improperly - of the Taoist tantric tradition in reference to the sexual teachings deriving from the doctrine of the Tao (in Chinese Dao = via).

In Taoism, esoteric sexual practices are the key kept secret for millennia to achieve prosperity, long life and immortality. The focal point of the practice is the retention of the male semen (also present in Indian tantra) to bring the man on an equal footing to the woman in the sexual sphere, and to achieve together the "rise of the Nectar (seminal essence) in the Flower of 'Oro (spiritual center on the top of the skull) ". The sublimation of the sexual energies, which "evaporate" in the body to reach the pai-hui (vertex of the head) and activate an energetic circle along the axial meridians, is a patient and methodical work of discipline accompanied by precise respiratory exercises, strengthening of the pelvic muscles, improvement of the creative visualization ability and focus of spiritual attention.

The way of the Tao is always a way in search of balance, in this case there is the harmonization of the external yin and yang (the woman and the man) and the internal yin and yang (in each lover), the result obtained is called "Double Elevation". Mantak Chia (master of Tai Chi, Qi Gong and sexual Kung Fu) has revealed to the West many of these ancient and secret practices, the diffusion of which could slow down that path of self-destruction undertaken by today's humanity and raise the spirit by safeguarding the energy resources. Chia defines his Tao Yoga method of love, the reading of his books is highly recommended for those wishing to learn more about the management of sexual energies, being clear, precise and extremely detailed texts.

The seven stages described by master Chia in progressing along the Taoist path of esoteric sexual practice are

- Physical (mechanical) domain of ejaculation
- Physical and mental domain of ejaculation
- Mental domain of the sexual impulse and orgasm
- Exchange of energy without sexual act
- Jing Chi mental elevation without partner and without self-stimulation
- Mastery in tapping into the yin and yang energies of the universe (extracorporeal dimension of the cosmic energy of the Tao)
- Achievement of immortality, final and complete union of the human being with the Tao.

Chapter 7: Tantric Sex And Tantric Sex Positions

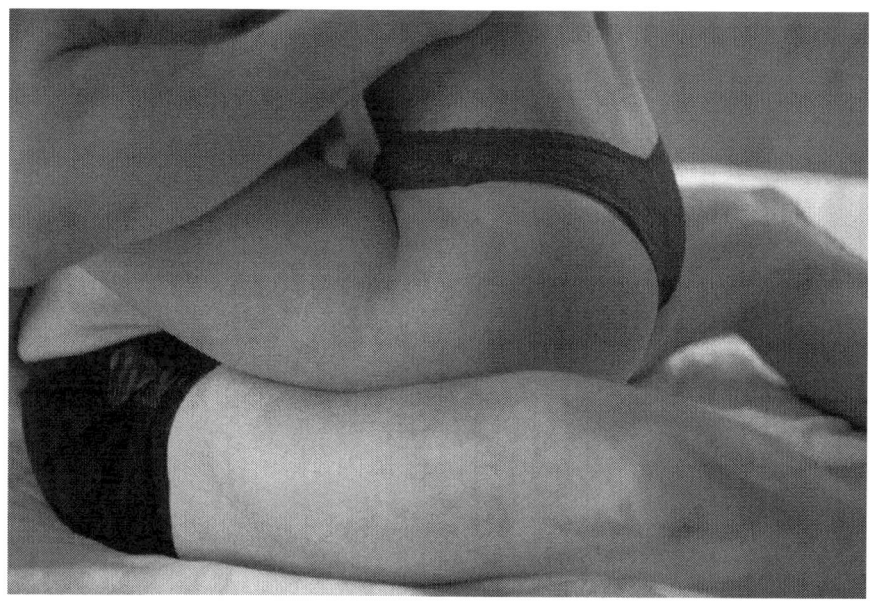

Tantric sex is an exclusive experience, a way of life, a view that has not too much in common with the sexual positions of the Kama Sutra. It enables the body and mind to liberate themselves and to experience intense and profound feelings of true bliss.

A practice started in India about 400 BC and its aim has continuously been self-knowledge and self-maturity. At that time, sexuality was in fact in use to connect to the other and to trigger the promoters of a person's nature. Over time, the term began to indicate that set of "sacred" sexual practices and rituals listed in tantric literature that allow the body and mind to free themselves and experience almost supernatural sensations. In today's society, where sexuality is experienced more with the head than with the body, tantric sex teaches the importance of slowness, attention, naturalness and complicity, all characteristics that deepen intimacy and increase passion , allowing you to communicate openly and authentically with your partner. Unlike customary sex, in tantric sex it is paramount to keep out the anxiety of orgasm, performance, result and in its place you must master to enjoy eroticism in its whole, from sounds to any other type sense and actions, scent, view, movements etc.

Who should go for Tantric sex

Tantric sex is more recommended for people who are particularly close since it is a more mental than physical practice that brings out all the psychological problems and motivations that underlie a relationship. At the same time, it is a practice that fights routine and allows you to create a deep, passionate connection, a real spiritual illumination. To face it in the best way, first of all you must not be afraid to try something new. Only with the mind and with the open heart will it be possible to reach total enjoyment. Subsequently, you must decide to dedicate at least one hour a week to your sexuality, even when you are tired or stressed. Tantric sex is in fact capable of invigorating the body and making it stronger and more energetic. In addition, the atmosphere is very important to reach the climax of pleasure: the bedroom must be a magical space, a temple of love, a real feast of the senses. It is therefore good to decorate the bed with pillows, blankets, flowers, incense and even some fruit and drinks. At this point, you can relax, removing any blockage or tension that prevents the body from experiencing deep and intense pleasure. In tantric sex, it is important to sit in front of the partner and meditate with him, connecting one's breath and heart with that of the other. Although it may seem strange practice, once you try tantra positions, the pleasure will turn into a real bliss. Tantric sex is a discipline also open to homosexuals, who can practice a sensual erotic massage for their partner. Such an intimate moment manages to rediscover one's body and achieve extreme pleasure. Homosexuality in the East has never been considered a taboo and it is precisely for this reason that such a passionate and intense sexual practice is open to all types of gender.

Tantric sex, the preparation

Many wonder if tantric sex really works. To make it an intensely erotic moment within the couple it is necessary to follow a series of "tricks". First of all, it is necessary to focus on your body and on the rhythm of the movement, in order to promote the circulation of energy. Voice emissions should not be blocked or inhibited for any reason. In tantric sex one must feel free to express one's pleasure at 100%. Finally, breathing deeply also helps to achieve pleasure. To improve the results, there are exercises to be performed together with the partner, so as to improve the entire sphere of sexual affectivity. For example, you can learn to breathe in the right way by using the diaphragm. You have to inhale for up to six seconds, hold your breath for another six seconds and exhale for another six. In addition, women must understand where the perineal area is, it can be used to stimulate orgasm only with the pelvic muscles, without any abrupt movement. The key to making tantric sex work is to listen to your body, reviewing its different parts and related sensations. These are the main guidelines you should follow when approaching Tantric Sex:

1. During tantric sex, physical contact is extreme, however the goal or goal is not to ejaculate or reach orgasm, but to experiment intensely every sensation, coordinate breathing and advance together with our partner to a higher level, in which exploration and the knowledge of the body through caresses and massages increases pleasure and interpenetration.

2. Since tantric sex is not an easy practice to do, it is recommended that you both have prior knowledge of meditation before you start practicing it. In this way, the basic aspects of this type of meeting, such as meditation and breathing, will already be clear to both.

3. To begin with you will have to choose a suitable place. Tantric sex in bed is not recommended, at least not in the early stages. The norm is to do it on the floor, properly made comfortable with a yoga mat or mat so that both of you are comfortable.

4. Perfuming the environment with incense or essences and lighting it in a soft way can help to achieve a good tantric sex encounter, stimulating intimacy and promoting meditation.

5. Once you are both comfortable and ready, exploration must begin. To practice tantric sex it takes time, so if you are in a hurry, the best thing is to postpone the meeting.

6. Start kissing, slowly and gently, then with intensity but without limits. Since tantric sex does not aim to achieve climax, kisses can be intense and unlimited in terms of time. The goal is union.

7. Caress your partner's body in its entirety, explore it totally from top to bottom with gentle but intense movements. Massages and caresses, using delicate objects such as feathers, are important in tantric sex.

8. Remember that the aim is to gradually acquire a greater ability to concentrate and to be able to feel good without quickly reaching physical pleasure.

9. Enjoy the sensations, but always stay focused on breathing, a fundamental aspect in tantric sex and meditation. You will have to continue to inhale and exhale during intercourse, not focusing solely on the sensations you perceive.

10. In the case of men, avoiding ejaculation during tantric sex is fundamental

11. Experience the ideal sexual positions for tantric sex to optimize results and be able to increase your stamina, in this way you will enjoy it more.

11. Do not expect that the first tantric sex meeting will reach a long duration. It is a gradual journey that requires concentration, meditation and patience to get results. Increase the fre-

quency of the meetings, work on concentration and breathing and you will see that improvements will come.

The must know Tantric sex positions

The positions of Tantra allow to improve the harmony in the couple's relationship and above all to rediscover a much more fulfilling, almost spiritual sexuality. The tantric positions refer to a precise oriental philosophy which foresees a reversal of the traditional male / female roles. The active part is the woman and has the task of transferring her "cold energy" to the male who transforms it into "hot energy". You don't want to orgasm but rather you want to increase your vital energy. The most known tantric sex position is where the woman sits on her partner's thighs, crossing her legs behind her back and holding him tight in a warm embrace. In doing so, you can also look him in the eye, creating a deeper connection.

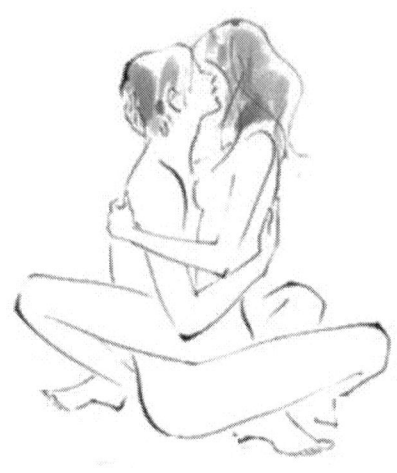

Another known position through the use a sufficiently high support, such as a table. The woman lies down and the man supports his legs on the sole of the foot, keeping them straight and perpendicular to the body. Muscle tension will increase the degree of excitement.

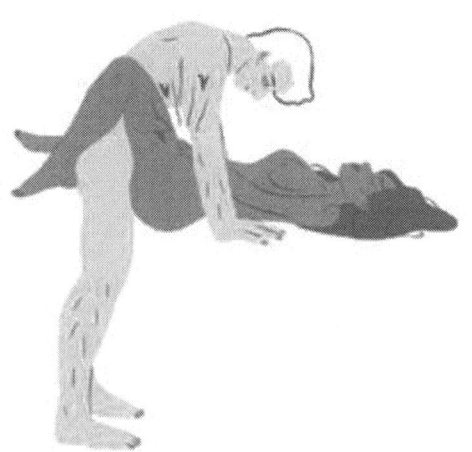

In the "hot chair" position, both partners are kneeling. The man stands behind his woman and pushes from behind, so that the two bodies are squeezed against each other tightly. Once the penetration has begun, the woman will have to make circular movements with her hips, taking regular breaks.

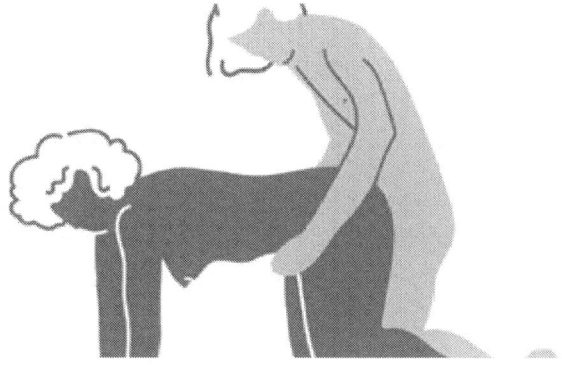

Other Tantric sex positions

The Fusion

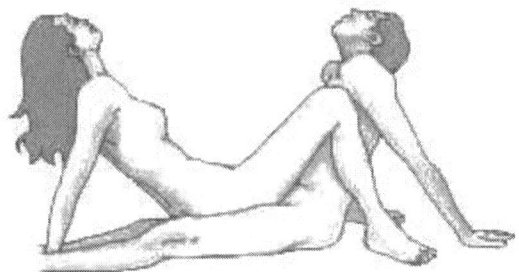

The Fusion is an excellent position for a tantric relationship, penetration is achieved slowly with circular movements, the act will always be slow, seeking control of sexual energy. This position is good for taking a break between kisses and caresses as it does not allow contact, only penetration and slow enjoyment.

The Missionary

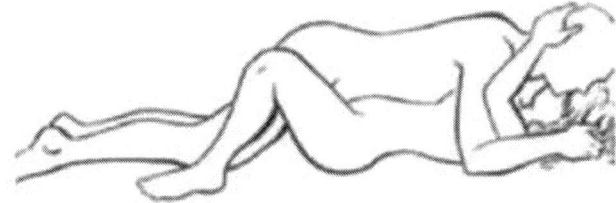

The missionary, a great sexual classic, is a good position for those who start tantric sex, since being the man who has control of the rhythm and penetration, he will be able to stop in time when he feels the desire to ejaculate, moving again to the kissing and caressing phase.

Fusion Variation

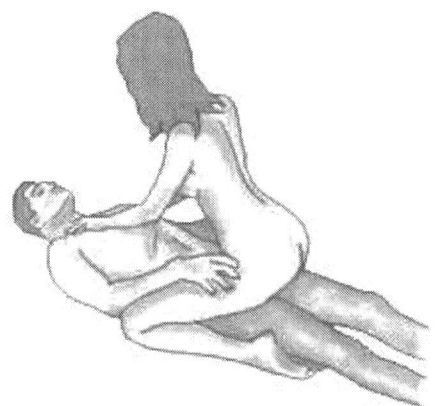

Another version of the fusion (which provides for greater contact between both), allows the woman to control the rhythm, making circular movements with the penis and feeling the flow of energy; however, this version requires human control to not reach orgasm earlier than desired.

The hug

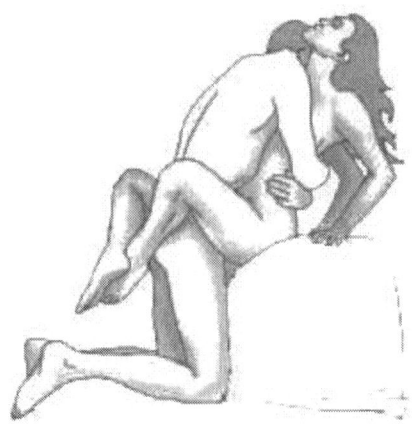

In this position, also the man manages to maintain control of the rhythm, also allows to caress the partner and this makes this position a very pleasant choice for both.

In tantric sex the positions are chosen based on preference: it is a matter of dominating the sexual energy of both and bringing enjoyment to the maximum point.

The Tantric chair and sex positions

The Tantra chair is a chair that has an ergonomic design that will help you make Tantra Sex Positions in a simple, safe and pleasant way. The sensual curves of the Tantra Chair are typically inspired by tantra wisdom and adapt perfectly to the curves of the body. Luckily, the 21st century is a time of full sexual liberty; hence there is no necessity to hide sex fantasies with your companion. Of course the Tantra chair can also be used for daily activities such as relaxing or reading. You can also take a nap or, if you prefer, work with the laptop.

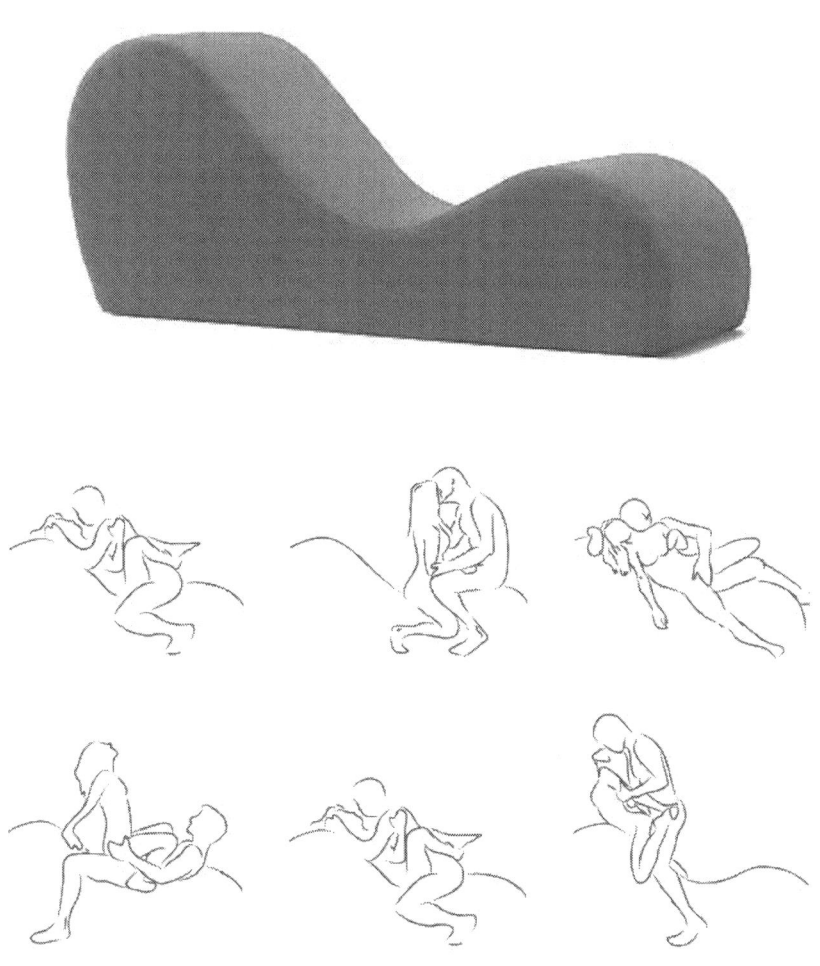

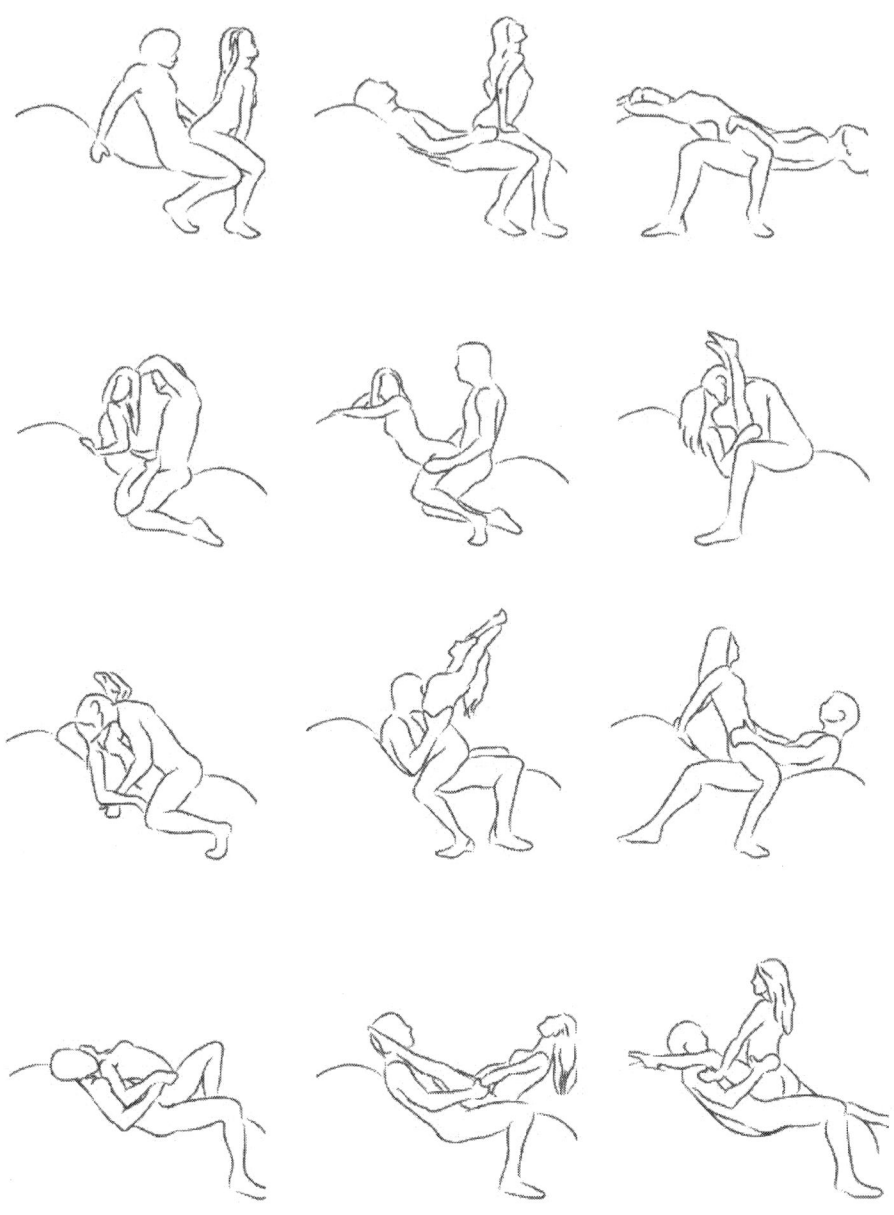

Tantric kiss technique

There are four basics steps to engage in tantric kiss:

1. Relaxation of facial muscle. Shut your eyes for a minute, breath as deeply as you can into your belly and let it out

2. Kiss your partner upper lips, using your both lips

3. Kiss your partner lower lips, using your both lips

4. Kiss your partner's both lips together.

Repeat and enjoy the energy building up.

Chapter 8: Tantric Massage

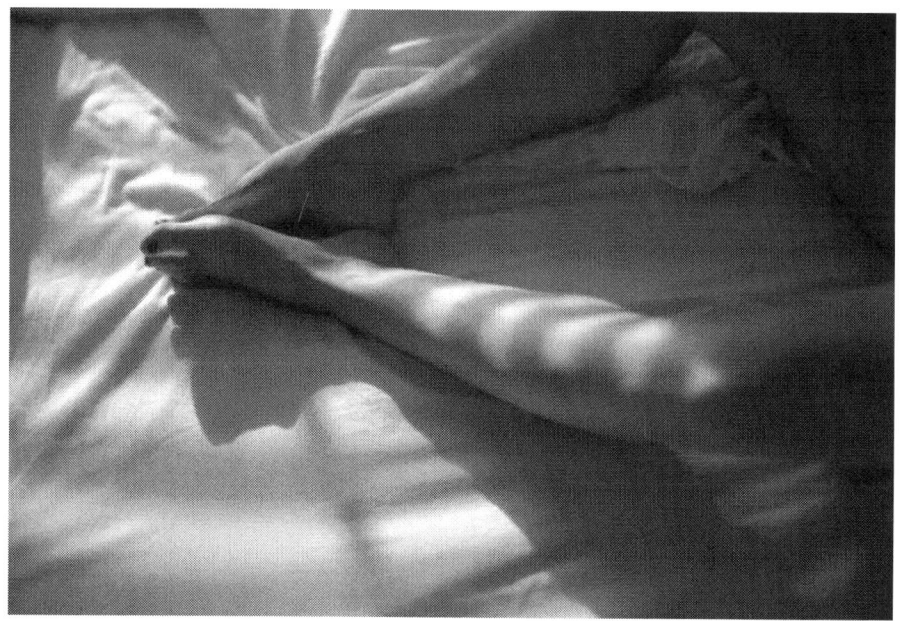

The basics of Tantric massage

The massage is among the deepest forms of exchange for both mankind and the animal world: most of the animal world participate in a seduction ritual that involves the gentle rubbing of bodies.

Generally, the Tantric Massage has the goal to bring to a physical experience of discovering the one-Self and, hence, of spiritual growth and vitality renaissance. When the person give the chance for a total admittance of himself/herself, to his/her real feeling beyond and away from schemes and social conditionings, there is an opening for access to more profound dimensions of Himself, so to be able to take full awareness and consciousness of who we really are in our totality.

In a more basic explanation, what actually distinguish the practice is the psychic aspect that is conveyed over an accurate focus which is taken to the "Heart" level and to the consciousness of the "Sacrality" of the body that hosts the Soul.

The term "tantric massage" therefore does not specify a determined structure or order, or specific manual abilities, but merely a method of massaging, a specific type of approach in the touching process. Basically, what describes a tantra massage is the "how" and not the "what".

Through the tantric massage and the stimulus of specific energetic points of the body, the individual that gets it feels a big sensorial enjoyment and at the same moment an enhancement of the self-perception of oneself and of one's own awareness. It is a great massage for the ones who want to intensify the knowledge and feel of agreement in the couple. Tantric massage is based on old Indian traditions, which goes back to manuscripts of ante-Vedic humanities, the original of which is left still rather enigmatic and contentious. The old Harappa population for instance, that millennia ago occupied some areas of India, considered of big meaning the energy produced by tantra, specially to the female character and its parts, water; in the middle of their homes there were usually large swimming pool and a chamber with a big bed on which to perform tantric massage.

It is not a basic erotic massage - as some people think - but a ceremonial in which all elements of the body are discovered and roused. The arms, back, legs, feet, the reproductive areas, the neck, the head and the face are - indeed - gratified with gentle pressure which relaxes and helps the respiration. This specific technique arrives from the East and has the goal of helping you find enjoyment and agreement of the senses. The Tantric massage is - for this reason - very indicated for couples, since it develops self-awareness - both for the ones who practice it and for the ones who receive it. The couple tantra massage is described as a spiritual ritual that joins the reciprocal wishes and feelings of the two persons involved.

If you do this massage in pairs, those who perform the massage give all their love to those who receive it. In the same way, the recipient completely abandons himself in the hands of the executor and prepares himself in a state of total trust. Really recommended for those who want to try a rapprochement with their partner in a time of strong stress or couple problems - especially sexual. By having a couple Tantra massage, you have the opportunity to discover something new about him/her. The approach takes place - in fact - both from a erotic and physical point of view.

What is Tantric massage best for

Doing or receiving a tantric massage enables you to reach the right equilibrium between psyche and body and to transfer this condition even in the act of love, for example with your partner / or, through the energetic release, so emotions are intensified you learn to control and prolong pleasure and the moments of ecstasy.

Tantra can help going over all that is hindered by our mental constructions, by our character, by our internal wounds, by our moral conditionings. A massage session is not to go too much into psychology, but simply support with the capability and consciousness of the current moment to get a more straight and clear understanding of the feelings of all our different bodily parts and to make us live the present better, "the now and the here".

The absence of flexibility in the physical body and mental attitude hinders the flow of energy: with the passage of time this block causes the acceleration of the aging process, the onset of physical diseases of various kinds and emotional issues ranging from depression to sense of guilt or general loss of love for life.

In the culture we live, all has got some form of construct from the greeting to the utmost private aspects, and it would be safe to assume that also many love interactions happen in a standard manner with recurrent and schematic actions, without any novelty and with limited mutual gratification. In the era of machines, humans are to be present in their physique, in their soul, mind, or spirit and emotions. Between these extremes, the handshake and the loving conjunction, there is today from the point of view of contact, a great void. If the feeling of loneliness is so widespread, the causes are to be found at least in part in this simple reality. The contact through the massage, when correctly applied, allows you to get out of the darkest labyrinth. The sweet and harmonious stimuli instill confidence. It is common knowledge that body contact cherishes self-confidence and the capability to believe, relax and let oneself go.

Effects of Tantric massage

Among the direct effects of tantric massage positive results can be found on the body, mental, and spiritual area, the decrease of stress, rigidities and energy reload, also transformations and alterations on the path of perceiving our being and the world that is around us, a rebirth of sexual drives may occur. Very frequently, those who get a tantric massage feel very neatly the revival or enhancement of body energy and creativeness.

Tantric massages are among the best ways to keep healthy and sustain a balanced nervous equilibrium in the constant discovery of our bodily parts. The curative part is surely a particularity of the tantric massage.

It also aims to encourage, where necessary, the unlocking of energy in a way that it streams freely through the body "meridians", affecting in a positive way all parts of life. In general, even where emotional blocks were not present, it enables for a progress in body vitality. The Tantric Massage can unlock energy and support in resolving the interior conflicts that affect the interpersonal relationship enabling you to have a joyful, healthy and rewarding couple experience; it can therefore also have beneficial effects on the couple, obviously if the couple can transcend aspects of jealousy and possession.

The Tantric Massage as we have already said can be though as a way of personal development like all other yogic practices as it enables a powerful physical experience, listening to one-Self, and liberating from conditioning. In practice, there have often been incredible beneficial effects on specific female and male problems connected with the psycho-corporeal sphere.

Skin is the thin layer dividing line between the inside and outside environment, and hands, as a mean to transmit and receive, are usually capable of entering into our profound, to trigger happiness and calm, to dissolve ties and rigidities, load it with vitality and if they are expert and sensitive enough, capable of feeling and feeling the other, they can also help the body's self-healing course.

The results, always important, are however individual and different from person to person and with different timing as always happens in any path of inner growth.

The results from tantric massage are not right away foreseeable, because its purpose is mainly to increase the person's hidden and unlocked energies. So, a priori, it is not possible to imagine what kind of energy will be expressed, if you like joy, emotion etc.

How Tantric massage should be performed

Tantric massage is consequently, in fact, a tantric practice. It occurs naked, both for the ones who receive and for the ones who give; Nudity brings to a more deep feeling in getting the massage, joint with a sense of greater freedom. At the time of the treatment, the body's energies are stimulated to move better, also augmenting enjoyment. All this helps to develop the awareness of one's senses, to get to know each other better both from inside oneself and relative to the external world.

It thus becomes a great opportunity for meditation and expansion of the Self through continuous listening. From a technical point of view, Tantric Massage is expressed through an intense succession of manual skills designed to stimulate a meditative state through a more intense perception of physicality and sensory abilities without also avoiding genital stimulation. In this case, the genital stimulation is not aimed at providing a mere pleasure, but at treating the genitals as if they were (and are) any other part of the body, without usually avoiding them morally, leaving this body part so important. It is the center of primary sexual energy, not integrated with the rest of the body, also because the tantra massage focuses on widespread body pleasure and not just genital pleasure. However Tantric Massage is not a method of implying an erotic relationship.

The human body is a totality and everything is sacred, worthy of attention. There are no areas closed by the Spirit. Unfortunately in our society, bad information and education is still widespread.

The deep meaning of massage is therefore of a global body integration which allows us to finally feel united and recomposed in the heart as well as in the perceived corporeality.

The Tantric Massage cannot be carried out in series, it will change and transform from person to person since everyone has a different body and energy. In addition, even performed on the same person, the massage will never be the same because the energy will change with it from time to time.

What type of sensations can the Tantric massage bring

Sensations and effects are entirely subjective, since it is a liberation of one's energy and a deep recognition of oneself and one's individuality, it is clear that perceptions and effects are varied. In general, however, it can be said that a constant sense of liberation, peace, harmony and rebalancing can be observed as constant effects.

It should be noted that Tantric Massage is not a standard technique that is learned in a book or on a videotape or worse in an online video course, but an expression of attention conveyed by Tantrika.

The Tantra massage can be carried out seriously only by those who are in the Tantric Way: someone who has realized the essence of tantra in their life. Tantra is experiential, it cannot be explained but only experienced and perceived personally. It cannot be studied, if anything, it can be a direct transmission; one could say a kind of 'initiation' that can only happen with particular Masters.

The spiritual aspect in tantric massage can be expressed through intimate and silent listening, inner purity, the action that comes from the Heart, the awareness of the "Sacrality of the body" perceived as the temple of the Soul.

The tantric touch is a tool that develops awareness that is the true and only goal of Tantra. The tantra ritual massage is both experiential and meditative, designed to awaken the body's consciousness by helping to reconnect with our unconscious where the traces of our most deeply rooted conditionings reside.

Tips on how to perform a Tantric massage

A Tantric Massage can be performed following three phases:

In the first phase we focus on meditation, creating a suitable and intimate place, such as the bedroom, a welcoming environment, with soft lights, incense, practicing exercises of breathing and reciting mantras.

The second stage concentrates on gentle and round massages that are done on the face and body, starting in the legs until the arms, going through the pubic area, the back, the neck and the head, with sweet touches along the channels of life energy, the chakras and nadis. A lukewarm and delicate carrier oil is used, such as coconut oil.

The last phase is relaxation: sipping a hot herbal tea shares the experience with those who have practiced it, verbalizing what has been tried.

The use of oil

Using essential oils for the body will make Tantra massage be even more effective and pleasant. This, in addition of an atmosphere full of incense and relaxing music. The oils good for tantric massage must be applied once you start to touch the recipient's body, and can be based on lavender, mint, calendula, basil, cinnamon, rosemary, sage, sandalwood, pine. Those are all fragrances known to stimulate blood circulation and promote muscle relaxation. Both for Tantra massage and for other types of oriental massages, essential oils are used since they have a strong penetration capacity in the body; in particular, coconut oil, which is aroma-free and does not irritate the skin.

How to make a Tantric massage to a woman – Yoni massage

The Yoni massage has recently gained some fans. The word Yoni, for those who do not know, has a Sanskrit origin and means the same as the female genital organ.

Some refer to the woman's vagina as a "sacred temple". This is because the vagina is a very erogenous zone and deserves to be explored in different ways, overcoming the spheres of oral sex and simple penetration. In the philosophy of Tantra, Yoni is considered with respect and love for followers.

The main goal of the Yoni massage is to make the woman deeply relax and experience sensations that she has never experienced in her entire life. In addition, the massage that is performed by men's fingers further extends the degree of intimacy between the couple, therefore essential for the health of the relationship. The partner of the massage is called "donor", to give the woman all the pleasure she deserves and should never expect anything in return.

Know that to do the Yoni massage in your partner you have to be selfless, you should never do the massage - which can also generate multiple orgasms in the woman and expect something in return or a pleasure. Sex after massage can also happen, but usually this is not the rule, especially if the woman enjoys and is already exhausted with so much pleasure.

Although this is not a sexual technique for men, it can be very pleasant for him, since he can see his partner as he has never seen before, trembling with so much heat and moaning like crazy. Which man has never thought of leaving a woman in this state, even with her powerful fingers? So learn the Yoni massage technique and apply it to your loved one!

Prepare the environment

Before you start, you must be careful to prepare the environment. In tantra, the place where sexual activities are given is very important, because it directly affects the whole process and the mental state of each. Putting a half light on the environment, smelling incense, flowers, lighting candles, arranging curtains, scarves and colored cushions can create a totally favorable atmosphere for what will come next.

Remember to put a silent ambient sound to balance the space. Humans are sensitive to the senses, therefore the activation of the sense of smell, hearing, sight and even touch can allow the experience to be more intense for the woman and increase her interaction with her. Even as a donor you will feel more relaxed in developing the technique.

First a nice shower

One of the recommendations of the Yoni massage is to take a relaxing shower before proceeding. The woman can bathe alone or you can participate in the bathroom by starting the ritual of connection and intimacy between you two. Try to make this moment something special, without haste and try to enjoy each other's presence. This bath will bring more vigor to both, as well as disinfect the entire region you will explore.

Balanced breathing

For the Yoni massage to work, it is important that your breathing is synchronized. Hence, man and woman should seek balance of breathing, a regular and calm breath. Shortness of breath shows insecurity, anxiety or even excitement in advance and the Yoni massage indicates that hormones are controlled and the woman is completely relaxed, available and confident with everything she will feel soon. Inhale and exhale together until you are in perfect harmony, if necessary you can also do a yoga session before finding the balance you need.

Disconnect from everything

You and your partner should be fully involved with each other and with the space they have prepared for the activity. Therefore, it is recommended to forget everything outside of that space all worldly and material things. Turn off the smartphone, notebook, close the door, unplug the intercom, the phone, close the windows, curtains and then immerse yourself in the universe you created. Obviously not only material matters are important, but you two should also make an effort not to disperse concentration with thoughts about problems and other concerns from outside.

Placement

Make sure to make the woman comfortable. You can let her observe the massage, the movements you perform and even your image, to make it even more stimulated. She may want to keep her eyes closed so that she can feel all the vibrations more fully, it will depend on the choice of each.

The legs should be separated and the knees bent in the typical position of a woman when she is about to give birth. Her genital organ must be fully exposed to you as a donor, who can sit in front of her to be able to perform all movements with ease and free access.

Start with the massage

Start by massaging her legs, thighs, breasts, abdomen and other regions before reaching the vagina. Pour a small amount of lubricant, which can be purchased in specialty stores and sex shops. Then squeeze the outer lip between your thumb and forefinger and slide up and down with slow and precise movements. Then, do the same movement on the inner lip, always calmly, getting the woman used to the touch. It is recommended that the couple maintains eye contact during the massage to intensify the sensation and the exchange between the two. Since the preference for intensity, speed and pressure varies from woman to woman, the woman should tell the donor what she prefers while experiencing the sensations. This will make it easier for the donor to find the right spot of pleasure. But try to limit the conversation, since prolonged speech can be a factor in dispersing the massage.

Focus on the clitoris

The clitoris is a complex structure, similar to the glans penis in the male sex. So it is extremely sensitive and erogenous, it can be up to four times more sensitive than the glans penis, in fact. This is because it has between 6 and 8 thousand nerves endings, which help to be one of the largest female pleasure generators.

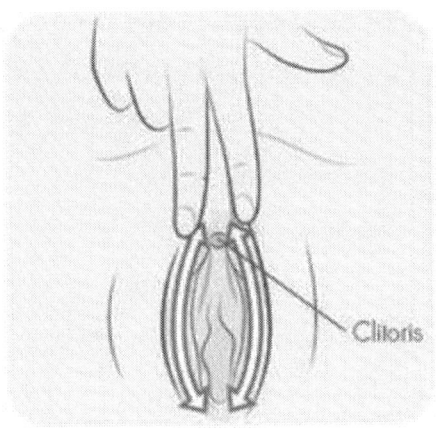

When massaging the clitoris, it is necessary to make circular movements clockwise and counterclockwise. Slowly insert the middle finger of your right hand into the vagina and make various movements - using your right hand has everything to do with the polarity of Tantra.

G-spot or "Holy Place"

Massage the inside of the vagina with your finger, varying the speed, depth and pressure. With your finger still inside the vagina, do the "come here" movement over and over again. In this area you will be in contact with a spongy tissue that is located under the public bone and behind the clitoris.

Finalization

At the same time you can use the little finger of the right hand to insert it into the woman's anus, obviously if she accepts. So, you can extend his feeling of pleasure with the Yoni massage. In the meantime, you can use your free hand (left hand) to massage the breast, abdomen or clitoris. The woman, completely sensitive to touch, can even cry due to the sensations, wince and have multiple orgasms. Just stop when she asks.

How to make a Tantric massage to a man

Unlike a conventional erotic massage, the tantric massage of the penis and lingam does not only aim to achieve ejaculation for your partner, but to stimulate energy of this important erogenous zone, to experience pleasure and to stimulate a sexual connection from a different perspective. Having made this philosophical-spiritual premise, let's go into more detail on how to do a tantric massage to a man.

1. To begin doing a tantric massage to a man, create an ideal environment for relaxation. Also, choose a moment of calm in which you know that you will hardly be interrupted because this massage will not be a quick meeting, so it is good that both participants immerse themselves in the moment without looking at the clock. Light up the house with aromatic candles

and incense. Create an atmosphere that promotes calm and pleasure.

2. Play to stimulate and excite your partner as you usually do, but relying on all your senses: your eyesight, stripping you gradually and seductively; touch, letting it caress your body and caress it in turn; the taste, with the flavor of kisses; the sense of smell with the smell of your lover's skin and yours and finally with hearing, thanks to a whole series of words and expressions of the erotic vocabulary that you know.

3. Before starting a tantric massage for a man, it is important to know all the sensitive points of your partner's genitals, as well as the whole penis. Stimulate the pleasure potential that can be obtained by stimulating the testicles, massaging the scrotum and stimulating the perineum, all extremely important areas for carrying out this massage.

4. Lubrication is essential for tantric lingam or penis massage. Use gentle oil like almond oil, which is a good conditioner that will give more delicacy to your movements making the experience a series of incredible sensations for him.

5. For this tantric massage you will have to use both hands, the movements will be ascending as indicated in the image and al-

so descending but in a more delicate way. One of your hands will massage the testicles, the scrotum and the perineum, while the other will focus on the penis from the base of the shaft to the glans, always keeping the rhythm and using your hands in their entirety. You have to take the penis and testicles with the whole palm, gently so as not to hurt, but confidently at the same time in order to generate pleasure.

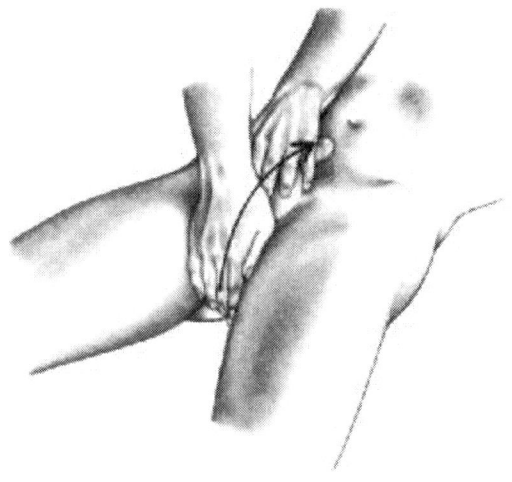

To do a tantric massage to a man, it is important that you let yourself go with pleasure in doing the tantric massage and infuse energy that your boy will perceive immediately. Try to be creative too, let the sexual energy permeate you to make your partner enjoy it too. Do not limit yourself, do not think if you are doing it well or badly, take advantage of this practice to increase intimacy and create new complicity.

Chapter 9: Tantric Yoga

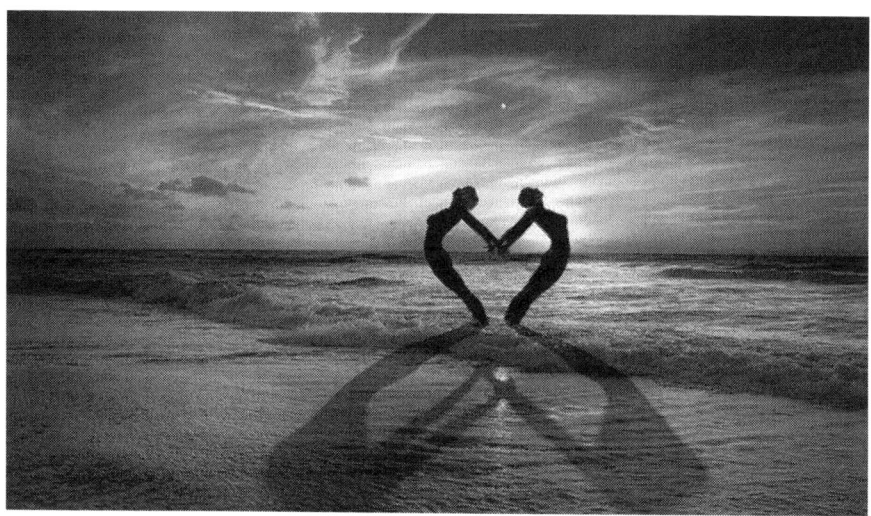

Despite what can be commonly heard, tantra yoga is a rather modern version of old traditions, which is slowly going through a process of clarification after a decade in which the tantra has speculated and has come to affirm all and the opposite of all. Tantra yoga, while in many of its forms does not differ much from hatha yoga. Among its goals, in addition to self-control, it includes the enjoyment of existence, in contrast to the liberation from the world desired by orthodox yoga. If for yogic belief the world is an artifice from which to liberate oneself (Maya), for tantra yoga it is a play of the Self (Lila) created for the own delight.

The different line of thoughts in tantra yoga

Before, tantric yoga was separated into two tracks, that of the left hand and that of the right hand, dakshina-marga and vama-marga. The path of the left hand alludes, probably metaphorically, to the use of erotic ritual as a yogic tool. The school of the right hand, less cryptic and not initiatory, centers on the kriya of purification of the being and the awakening of the kundalini, in order to empower the understated bodies and thus allow the spiritual to connect to the body. Tantra yoga today is quite close to hatha yoga, based mainly on asanas to be done in couples, on meditative practice and for the use of mantras and mudras. If it is correct that many count among the benefits of tantra yoga as an improvement in sex life, this does not necessarily indicate that sex is seen as one of the means of tantra yoga. Tantra yoga, supports in bringing liveliness and success into life overall, as well as economic and social life, if needed. In its practice none of the existing bodies according to the tantric tradition is neglected:

- the carnal body is kept uncontaminated and healthy
- the physique energy is purified thanks to mudras, mantras and respiration workouts so as to allow the energies to flow
- the psychological body is made silent and receptive to intuitions

- the soul is placed at the helm of the entire being
- the physique of heaven, the anandamaya purusha, is enabled and activated, therefore able to live bliss in the actions of all the other bodies.

Tantra yoga key exercises

Much significance is given to positions in pairs and to the stream of vitality and feelings that come from these positions.

1. Synchronized breathing

The best way to start this experience for two is to breathe in unison. Sit cross-legged and position yourself back to back. Close your eyes, concentrate on the rhythm of your partner's breathing and try to adapt.

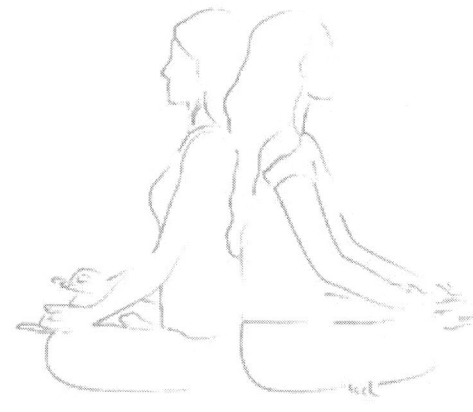

2. Twisting in pairs

Sitting back to back with your legs crossed, synchronize your breath and turn your torso to the left, then rest the back of your left hand on your right knee and your right hand on the partner's knee.

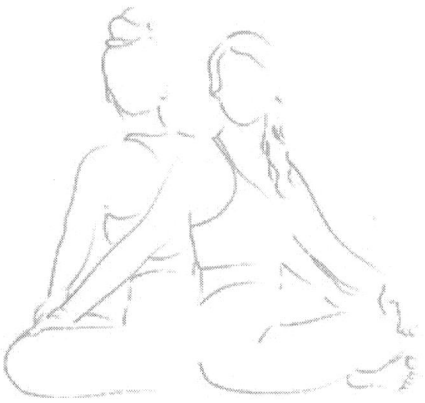

3. Position of the boat

Sit on the ground, at a distance that allows you to grasp each other's wrists by stretching your arms. Bend the legs and place the soles of the feet close to those of the partner, then extend and raise the legs.

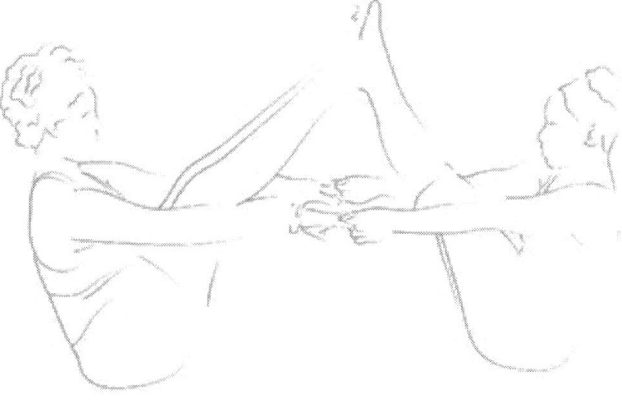

4. Ripple movement

Sit back to back with your legs crossed. One of the two flexes forward until he draws his chest against his legs, while the partner follows his movement arching backwards and abandoning himself on his partner's back.

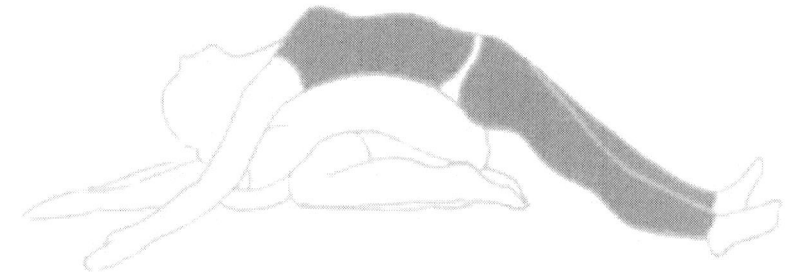

5. Standing forward bend

Standing forward bending, or Uttanasana, can be done in pairs. Standing, back to back, raise your arms, contract your abdomen, bend your back forward and bring your hands to the floor. Then try to grab the partner's shoulders and look each other in the eyes upside down.

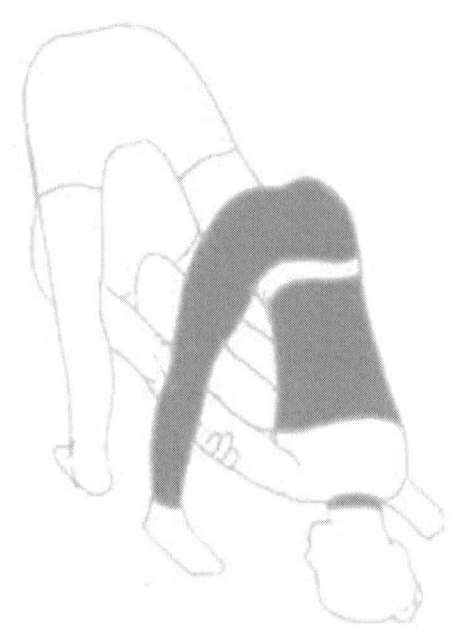

6. Tree Pose

Stand next to each other and wrap your "inside" arms around your partner's waist. Use your "external" arm (if needed) and tweak your "external" leg upwards to make a tree position. When you have reached balance you can either connect each other's hands in a Namaste hand position or on top of your head as in a moon position.

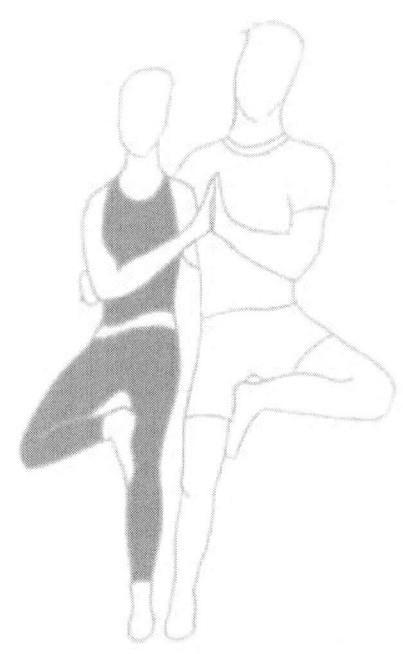

7. Wide Angle Sitting Forward Bend

Sit down and wide open the legs as comfortably as you can. Let companion sit in front of you and have their feet either above your ankles or below your knees. Move yourself onward as far as you can make it. If more comfortable, you can let your partner take your forearms (between your wrists and elbows) and softly pull yourself near your partner.

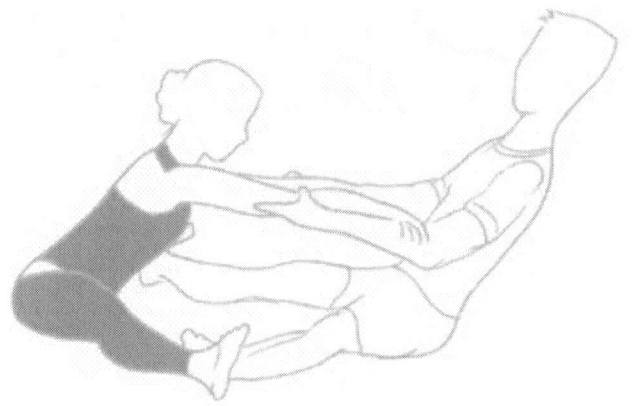

Other exercises go into more private type of contact, but it is good to underline one thing. Many tantra yoga teachers claim that while this practice contemplates orgasm, there is not much sexual around it. Tantra yoga arrived in the West exactly in its moment of rebellion against the oppressive educational norms and with all the counterculture that pushed to the liberty of the body and its usage. At the time, therefore, this discipline took a misleading path and often many have undertaken it in the anticipation of finding their own cravings. But tantra yoga teaches us that orgasm is already intrinsic in each of us. There is no necessity for sex, there is no necessity for a mate and it can be practiced in every part of the body, even in the peripheries such as the fingers and the head and this is possible only by becoming aware of one's own body energy.

Chapter 10: Feminine Orgasms And Tantra

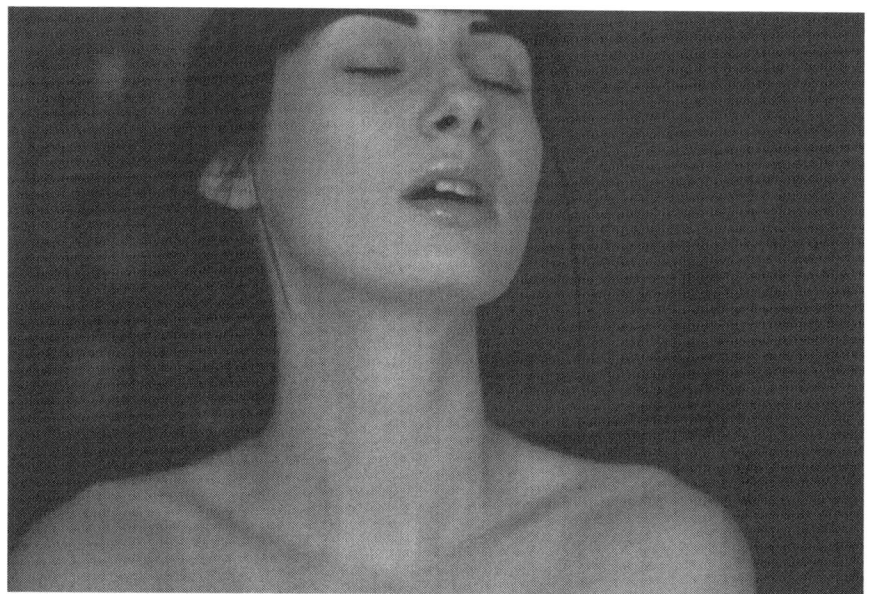

In the moment of orgasm the woman experiences the state of maximum abandonment and this type of experience can be expressed each time in different ways in a kaleidoscopic universe of pleasure. If the man had a remote control for pleasure it would have only two buttons, on and off, while the woman's remote control would be equipped with various buttons that vary according to the emotional state, the moment and the situation.

Explosive orgasm and implosive orgasm

Although the orgasmic experience of the woman may involve various erogenous points simultaneously in a cocktail of sensations that are not easily defined, we can still make an initial distinction between:

Explosive orgasm, superficial experience that involves the dispersion of energy outside the woman's body. It only involves the genital area and the lower chakras (first and second), often leaves a sense of tiredness and frustration because it does not bring complete contentment. Clitoral orgasm is of this type.

Implosive orgasm, experience in which the energy does not disperse outside but implodes inwards and towards the upper chakras. It can involve the whole body, as well as the mental and emotional spheres of the woman, giving a deep state of fulfillment, physical, mental and emotional. The vaginal orgasm and the cervico-uterine orgasm are of this type.

Clitoral orgasm

There are many women who, for now, have not found the way to orgasm and others manage to reach only that through the clitoris (however already an excellent starting point). The clitoral orgasm, despite still being an incomplete and superficial experience, shows the woman that ocean of pleasure that is already inside her. It reveals the orgasmic nature of every woman, but it would be a real pity to stop at this level and be content with the more superficial layers of pleasure.

Explosive orgasms start from the clitoris, which involve, like male ejaculation, the dispersion of vital potential and also develop an energy that remains at the level of the lower chakras, often leaving a state of hyperemotivity, tiredness, or other unpleasant feelings.

The woman could spend her life thinking she is a "clitoral" and that she cannot do anything about it. It is important to know, however, that almost every woman can have access to deeper and more satisfying levels of pleasure. Tantra teaches that all women can experience internal orgasm, following a path of awareness of their body and their physical, mental and emotional blocks.

Vaginal orgasm

When an orgasm also involves the internal walls of the vagina, then we can speak of internal orgasm, which by its nature is implosive. Many women who are accustomed to external orgasm remain displaced in front of the experience of deep orgasm: the former is mainly concentrated on the genitals, while the latter is widespread, expanded, enlarged to the whole body.

This type of experience gives a sense of deep emotional fulfillment. Although it is often accompanied by the expulsion of a large amount of liquids, it does not involve dispersion of energy, but rather the woman feels energetic, luminous, sensual and is ready to experience another orgasm of even greater intensity.

A few centimeters from the entrance of the vagina, along the front wall of the vaginal canal, there is the famous "G-spot". It is made up of erectile tissue, therefore it swells when it is sexually excited and only then it can be perceived by touch, as a more sensitive area.

Orgasm at the "G-spot" level is often perceived as a pleasant sensation of electric shock that expands from the vagina into the abdomen, along the arms and head. Energy implodes upwards, flooding the chest, changing the breath and accelerating the heart, in an experience of deep emotional transformation.

For many women, the stimulation of the "G-spot" is too intense or even painful and they prefer to avoid touching it, both during masturbation and during intercourse with their partner. By continuing to explore the area, however, and gently stimulating it, the nuisance will slowly dissolve to make way for an ocean of pleasure that involves the whole body.

This process may take time and practice to open up the full potential of the "G-spot" and the sensations of deep orgasm, especially for women who have lived until now completely ignoring it. The best way to access this type of orgasm is to train through the use of a Yoni Egg or Vaginal Egg.

Cervix-uterine orgasm

In the pantheon of woman's sexual experiences there is an even deeper erogenous point that resides at the level of the cervix, that is, the area where the vagina opens into the uterus.

The orgasm that arises from the cervix is manifested by deep slow vibrations of the vaginal musculature that rise up to involve the wall of the uterus, for this reason it is called cervico-uterine. This is the tantric orgasm par excellence. There are not many women who reach this incredibly deep type of orgasm, but those who discover it would not change it for anything in the world. All of them express an incredible change: a process of profound transformation takes place in the most subtle levels, something changes at the level of the mind and emotions, something opens and blooms. Taking full contact with their sexual power, they become bright and beautiful, they seem to shine with their own light.

Deep penetration is required to stimulate the cervix. Sometimes these points can be a little painful, especially if they have never been stimulated, other times they can be turgid or numb. During the penetration ask your partner to gently touch your deepest points, move the pelvis to find the right angle that allows him to get to the bottom. At the beginning you may feel a sense of annoyance or a slight pain, but continue the same asking him to be delicate and breathe trying to relax the abdomen. Welcome any kind of sensation that springs from within your body.

With a gradual and sweet approach, the initial annoyance will disappear to make room for the most intense and deep pleasure. If you don't have a partner, you can treat yourself to a self-massage with a special tool. When you get a taste for deep penetration, you will only look for that one as it is much more satisfying, until you disclose the experience of tantric orgasm.

For an instant only there can be the perception of an incredible state of abandonment until the cancellation of time, the mind ceases the continuous production of thoughts and for a moment there is a state of mental emptiness, the boundaries of one's being expand and the energy field increases.

The tantric orgasm, an extraordinary experience

For thousands of years in the discipline of Tantra, the link between orgasmic sexual experiences and states of expansion of consciousness has been discussed, opening a solid bridge between sexuality and spirituality.

Sometimes the experience can be so intense to the point that you get to perceive yourself in a state of fusion of your ego with something bigger, of a cosmic whole. This experience is comparable to what in Yoga is called Samadhi, in Satori Buddhism and which the Christian Saints call Mystical Union.

The ultimate state of spiritual realization has been described by the mystics of all centuries as the fusion of the individual microcosm with the universal Macrocosm, accompanied by an indefinable pleasure, beyond any mental understanding. It has also been called Cosmic Orgasm.

The best way to access this type of orgasm is to train through the use of a Yoni Egg or Vaginal Egg.

Chapter 11: The Yoni Egg

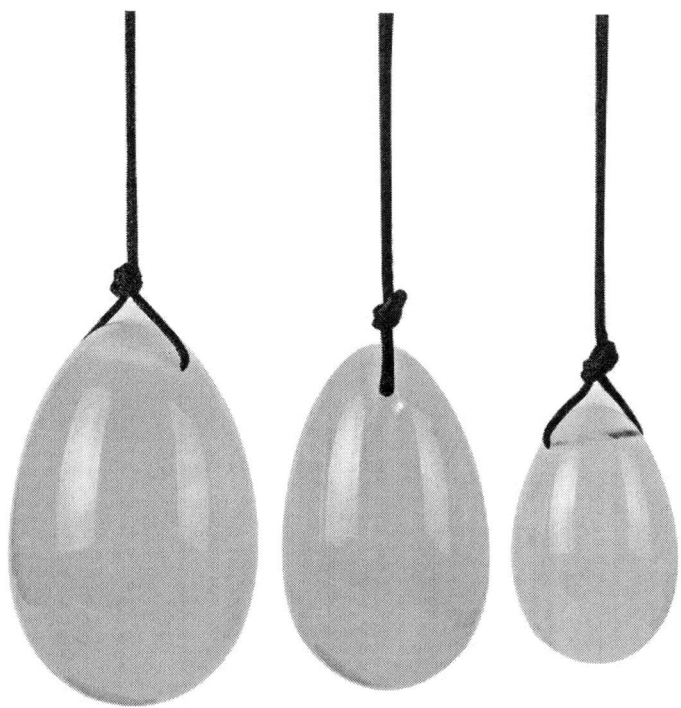

Origins of the Yoni egg

The relationship between the condition of the vagina and the general state of physical and mental health of the woman was also well known in ancient China, the cradle of wisdom in which Chinese Medicine originated, the oldest medical system in the world.

The practice of Yoni egg also known as Jade egg was secretly passed down and kept only for the emperor's wife and concubines, who used it regularly to train and regenerate the vaginal muscles, in order to please their sovereign in the bed arts. It was thus possible to see how much these women maintained a general state of health and energy even over time.

Already 3000 years before Christ, Jade was considered precious in China and was called "the royal stone" for its many beneficial properties. It was also called the stone of long life, mental clarity, emotional balance. It was believed to provide protection against physical ailments and adversity, rebalance the nervous system and was considered a source of wisdom and sincerity. Confucius defined it as "the mirror of the integrity of the soul".

Benefits of the Yoni egg

- Tones the pelvic floor muscles, therefore helps prevent urinary incontinence and uterine and bladder prolapse
- It increases passion, libido and creative energy
- It increases awareness of the vaginal wall, improving its sensitivity
- Increases orgasmic capacity

- Bringing vaginal walls back together, so it is useful after pregnancy and childbirth (but also for partner's happiness)
- Improve the couple's understanding
- Improve vaginal lubrication
- Prevents dysmenorrhea (excessive menstrual pain)
- Rebalances hormonal life at every age of the woman
- It reduces menopause-related ailments, such as vaginal dryness and hot flashes
- Brings harmony on an emotional level
- It removes energy blocks and psychological traumas, improving the relationship with one's sexuality.

Types of Yoni eggs and how to get one

It is possible to buy a Jade egg through specialized sites on the internet, where Yoni Egg of various minerals such as Rose Quartz, Obsidian, Amethyst or others are commercially available. For those who begin the practice, it is recommended to buy one of real Jade, for its immense energy and therapeutic properties, known for millennia.

Please pay special attention as Jade is a fairly rare mineral and therefore often mistaken for a lighter stone called "new jade" or "serpentine", light green in color. The real Jade is instead of dark green color.

Be careful to buy and use only Eggs that are sold specifically for intimate practice: often, during the processing of decorative hard stones, chemicals, dyes or artificial fillers are used that make the stones brighter and more colorful, but not safe to use for this intimate and sacred practice. Make sure to buy only Yoni Eggs created with natural and certified stones and crystals to be used in contact with the Yoni.

Once you have got your Jade egg, you need to clean it thoroughly, especially the first time. It is enough to boil it in water, remove it from the heat, wait for it to cool down and immerse the egg in it for 5 minutes. If desired, one or two drops of tee tree oil or lavender essential oil can be added to the water. It is better not to boil Jade directly in order not to damage its properties, and to avoid the use of chemical disinfectants or soaps that could leave traces on its surface and irritate the delicate vaginal wall.

A common fear of women who begin to use the Jade Egg is the fear that, once inserted, it will get lost inside the vagina. This fear is completely unfounded! The vaginal canal is closed at the bottom by the cervix, so there is no danger that the Yoni Egg will rise higher.

To avoid this apprehension, however, it is possible to buy an egg with a hole at its smaller end, so that you can insert a wire. Dental floss can be used, inserted double in the small hole, so as to create a loop in which the other end of the thread can be inserted creating a knot. In this way we will have secured the egg to the wire that will remain outside the vagina during use. We will then proceed to use our Jade Egg without the fear that it will get lost inside the body.

Which Yoni egg size to use

Many women naturally have a large vagina, even regular sexual activity and any natural parts can enlarge the vaginal canal; in this case a larger egg may be needed.

Through intimate gymnastics with the support of the egg, the vagina will regain the width of when you were a girl and then you can switch to a smaller egg.

You can also buy sets of three eggs of different sizes: the largest of the size of a normal chicken egg, one medium and one even smaller. Beginners will start with the bigger ones and gradually move on to the smaller ones.

Do not be alarmed if, despite you are using a large Yoni Egg, you do not perceive any sensation: simply take note of the fact that your vagina needs to be toned and activated. Arm yourself with willpower and promise yourself to do the exercises every day.

How to use the Yoni egg

Create the ideal situation for such an intimate practice, avoiding to do it in a hurry. Take the time to prepare the room, light a candle, put on music that relaxes you and makes you feel good. Lie on the bed and stretch your whole body to ease the tensions, take a couple of good deep breaths.

The first precaution to have is to heat the Jade to the temperature of our body. We could hold it in our hand for a little while, or we could put it between our clothes and the skin at the level of the abdomen or belt.

The ideal condition would be that our vagina was naturally moistened. Before inserting our magical egg let's take the time to feel the body, caress and give us a breast massage to stimulate the hormonal reaction that will lubricate the vagina. Breast massage is a very healthy practice for the mammary gland, it also helps to relax psychic tensions. However, it is possible to use a lubricant such as sweet almond or coconut oil.

Once the egg is inserted, it brings awareness to the yoni (from the Sanskrit "sacred temple", is the term with which the vagina is called in the tantric tradition) and listens to all the sensations you perceive.

The mere fact of keeping the Jade egg in the yoni for a few hours will significantly increase the sensitivity of this remote area of the body. A large series of nerve endings will be stimulated so as to create new neuronal connections between the brain and the vaginal wall, starting a new awareness process.

Many women do not have complete vaginal sensitivity and consequently their sexual relations are not satisfactory enough, due to a dissociation between the brain and the erogenous points in the vagina. This situation can be quickly transformed by starting to bring more attention to this area. The Jade egg is an excellent ally for this purpose.

When to use the Yoni egg

If you keep the egg in your body while walking, cleaning the house, dancing, practicing yoga, your vagina will maintain a slight contraction so that the egg does not come out due to the effect of gravity. In this way you will train the muscles of the vaginal walls, while the movement of the egg inside will create a constant and pleasant yoni massage, relaxing unnecessary tensions.

If in the upright position the egg tends to come out easily, even if you try to contract the muscles, your yoni is telling you that she is down in tone and that she needs a little gym.

If, on the other hand, you find it difficult to insert the egg because the vagina is closed or you cannot relax it enough to make it come out, then your flower is telling you that it is tense and contracted and that you must teach it to relax.

Kegel's contractions

To have the maximum muscle toning effect, you should combine Kegel's contraction and relaxation exercises:

Once the Yoni Egg is inserted, try to contract the vaginal muscles so that it goes up along the canal, then relax until you feel it come down. Repeat the contraction several times, starting with 10-20 up to 150 cycles per day.

Remember to always end with adequate relaxation of the muscles and not to overdo the number of repetitions. Always proceed very gradually to create the result of a strong but also soft and elastic perineum. You are working with the "sacred temple" of your body, sweetness and sensitivity are essential attitudes for such a delicate, feminine and vulnerable area.

It is essential to start gradually, keeping the egg in the vagina for one hour a day. If you feel discomfort or pain during this time, you can remove it (but this happens very rarely).

Then increase according to your feeling. Over time, some women insert it in the morning when they go to work and keep it indoors all day, others love to insert it at night because they have noticed an effect on the quality of dreams.

It is good to follow your instincts, listen to yourself and guess what the right time is for you, without falling into unnecessary exaggerations that could create counterproductive tension and rigidity.

Effects from using the Yoni egg

The effect of jade at the level of the second chakra produces a profound energetic purification, which translates into the harmonization of emotional plans. For this reason many women who use the yoni egg report feeling a lot of inner calm and psychological balance.

The practice with the jade egg helps to become aware of one's deep erogenous points and turns out to be a valid aid to increase vaginal sensitivity. Toning the vaginal muscles improves the quality of the internal orgasm which will become incredibly deep and satisfying, eliminating tension and stress from the body and mind, and opening the woman to the maximum creative potential in all areas of life.

To open oneself to the maximum orgasmic potential goes far beyond from merely feel pleasure, it is to find a deep physical and spiritual fulfillment, to move and channel the energies to open oneself to deep ecstatic states that open to spiritual dimensions.

The practice of the egg is particularly suitable for removing energy blockages due to past traumas, which can remain stowed in the cellular memory of the vagina, uterus and cervix.

Unpleasant, emotionally unbalanced or even traumatic sexual experiences can leave a bad memory in the body of a woman, especially at a young age and can affect the relationship with one's sexuality and femininity for a long time.

Penetrations too early, when the yoni was not yet ready, or violent, lacking the space of sweetness necessary to become open and receptive, not to mention violence, where the vagina is violated without the woman's permission, can create permanent anxiety of penetration, the tremendous fear of opening up and letting go.

The practice of the jade egg can be a valuable aid to dissolve these energy blocks and cause energy to start flowing again where it was blocked, and thus improve the relationship with themselves.

Chapter 12: Pompoir For Men, How To Control Ejaculation And Last Longer

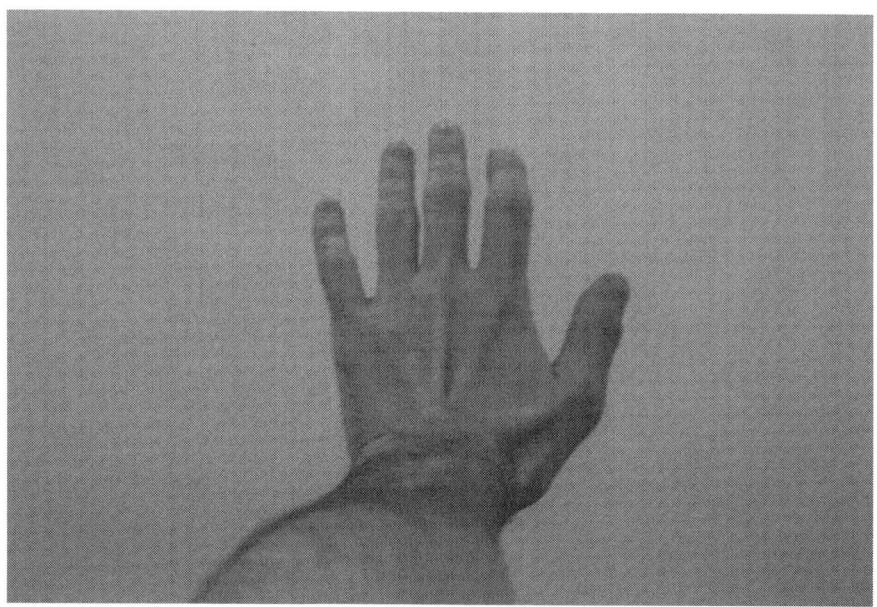

Also men want more pleasure. Which man wouldn't want to take more than two in a row, prevent impotence and increase the quality of the orgasm?

Pompoir is a set of techniques of oriental origin, used to strengthen and control the muscles of the vagina, usually to increase sexual pleasure. Known widely for its benefits for women, the word Pompoir derives from the Tamil language, spoken in Sri Lanka and southern India, and means mental command over the pubococcygeus muscle, the circunvaginais muscles and the large labia of the female vulva. But in this chapter we will see how to do some specific exercises for men that will help increase self-esteem, virility and self-control.

What is Pompoir for men

Who does not want to reach deeper orgasms, increase pleasure and prevent disease. These are some of the benefits offered by Pompoir and you will learn the basics here to start having more pleasure and lasting longer.

This sexual gymnastics known by select groups of people in India, Thailand, Indonesia and other Eastern countries has spread all over the world. This technique has been developed by these people for over 1,500 years.

Although it is usually associated with women the ancient art of Pompoir can also be practiced by men. It promises to expand the quality of sexual life and hot moments together. Pompoir for men is the technique of intimate gymnastics based on regular exercises that help to improve coordination, skill and muscle strength.

These exercises bring highly significant results to the health of your sexual organs. Increasing your self-knowledge, control, you will know exactly when to stop stimulating, before that point of no return.

Often, speaking of male Pompoir, reference is made to a version close to the female, which includes the introduction of some tools in intimate parts for the development of the practice. But in practice male Pompoir has nothing to do with it.

The exercises are performed only by stimulating the muscles, contracting and relaxing, and there is no reason to worry about. Forget the idea of Pompoir as something feminine and understand all the benefits that this practice can generate for your sexual and daily life.

Male Pompoir is the key to extreme pleasures. To achieve these goals, be patient and kind to yourself, some of the exercises listed below can be reconciled with some daily activities such as driving, sitting in the office, watching TV and, of course, during sex.

Benefits of Pompoir for men

The benefits of male Pompoir are to strengthen the pelvic region, leading to greater blood circulation, allowing man to have sex for hours, maintaining a stiff erection, controlling ejaculation and feeling more sensitive. This will make the man last longer and get better orgasms.

For men, the act of Pompoir brings several benefits with practice. First, there is an improvement in sexual performance, that is, the man, in addition to lasting longer, has more vigor. This happens due to the strengthening of the pelvic muscles and the improvement of blood circulation, which increases the effects of erection.

In addition, the exercises ensure greater control of the region, including with regard to stimuli and ejaculation time. A man who practices male Pompoir tends to suffer much less with premature ejaculation than others.

The practice also promotes control of other activities, such as attention to breathing and self-knowledge. They may seem small factors, but they are absolutely important for the development of a higher quality of life.

How to start practicing Pompoir for men

First, you should start with adequate breathing throughout the practice. For this, it is important to inhale deeply through the nose. Do this with your abdominal muscles relaxed. Exhale slowly, still through the nose, making sure that the movements are always concentrated in the abdomen.

This perception is essential for the control of the body. It allows the diaphragm to be responsible for breathing, which makes the body function properly, without disturbing the muscles to be worked on during the exercise.

The target muscles of male Pompoir are the pubococcygeus muscles. They are located between the male penis and the anus and are the same muscles used, for example, to stop the flow of urine when in the bathroom.

Exercises for the Pubocoxigen

First Exercise - Also known as Kegel Exercise

When urinating, try to contract the muscles to stop the urine flow, repeat it several times. It is normal during the first attempts to feel a burning sensation. If you are able to stop the flow it means that you are on the right track. But don't go overboard.

Second exercise - Muscle knowledge

Sitting in a comfortable place with your spine erect, try to contract the muscle you used to stop the flow of urine. Well, now focus on that region and do short and fast contractions, start with 10 reps and gradually increase. Note that your penis will move during contractions. It is normal for the belly and anal muscles to contract initially, but over time, you should only be able to contract this muscle. Do 3 reps 10 times a day.

Third exercise: movement control

Standing and naked in front of a mirror, contract the pubococcygeus several times and observe the movements of the penis. The stronger the muscle, the stronger the movements of the penis.

Thank you!

The End

Made in the USA
Middletown, DE
07 November 2020